wards, offices, and, yes, on the battlefield are rarely mentioned in the history books, at least those commonly read outside the profession. The nurses I met and interviewed were women in the ranks—in every sense. They were middle-class; married, divorced, or single; childless, or members of suburban PTAs; committed to an ambitious career plan, or working to help pay the mortgage. Some were committed to their profession, their *calling*. Others saw nursing simply as a way to make a living.

Looking back today, I can say there was really nothing remarkable about the women in my study. They were not smarter or braver or stronger than other women I had known. But they were different, somehow wiser, or so it seemed to one who had not "been there," as some of them used to say. A decade or two ago they went off to war and many of them performed their jobs well under the worst of conditions, so many in fact that they dispelled the common notions about women's stamina, mettle, and endurance. They did not come home hardened and insensitive; they came home confident that no future test would be as difficult as the one they had just passed.

At first, I thought it would be easy to find them. In this era of overzealous record-keeping, I assumed I could call someone in Washington, D.C. and obtain a list. I checked with the Army, Navy, and Air Force Nurse Corps, the army nurse historian, the air force nurse historian, the Veterans Administration headquarters, the public information services at the Pentagon, the American Nurses Association, the National League for Nurses, and Vietnam Veterans of America. No one had a list. "We never thought it a record of nurses' statistics was important to keep," a researcher at Water Reed Army Hospital said.[2] An army general wrote, "The problems of obtaining an unbiased sample are real."[3] In effect, nobody knew who or how many nurses served in Vietnam.

Their names and accomplishments are a matter of record but the records are among the millions of names in the National Personnel Records Center, Military Division. All Vietnam veterans, both male and female, are listed there. Each is identified by a service number or social security number, and by military occupation. Even if the Privacy Act could be waived, it was unrealistic to think that anyone could effectively cull those records to put together an accurate list. Moreover, no one could say how many names would be on such a list. Estimates of the number of military nurses who served in Vietnam range from 4,000 to 15,000. A 1985 newsletter published by the Vietnam Veterans of America put the number at 11,000.[4] But this figure includes all military women in Vietnam, not just nurses.

Why the poor record-keeping? There were two reasons. First, military nurses were not considered a significantly large group to necessitate separating them out from all of those who served. No one thought that researchers would be interested in this group after the war. The veterans themselves kept in touch with only a few of their friends. They tried to blend back into society. They had little interest in trying to find an old comrade from their former hospital or air evacuation group and little interest in big reunions. In the years when these women went to war—1965 to 1973—feminism had not yet taken hold. Women in large numbers had not yet reawakened. There was not much call for information about military nurses and certainly not much interest in this group. No one, in fact, began to ask for information or lists until the early 1980s, when controversies like the Agent Orange issue appeared.[5]

I found the nurses who appear in this book by use of a research technique called "snowball sampling." People I worked with in New Jersey and people I studied with at New York University gave me the names of four nurses who met the qualifications I had set for participants: they had to be women, registered nurses, members of the Army, Navy, or Air Force Nurse Corps, and veterans of Vietnam. I asked the first four women I interviewed for the names of other nurses. This process of obtaining names continued until I had completed fifty interviews. Those interviewed were selected from a list I developed of 122 women who had served in the military as nurses in Vietnam. All women interviewed lived or were visiting the East Coast. There were no research grants for my study and no money for travel.

The women in this study served in Vietnam from 1965 to 1973. They worked in over thirty different hospitals, ships, and airfields in South Vietnam. They were fairly evenly divided between those still in the military and those who are now civilians. The majority were in the Army Nurse Corps, the largest nursing

Given to
Wayne Erwin

Women at War

By Doughter
Laura Estep

Christmas
2005

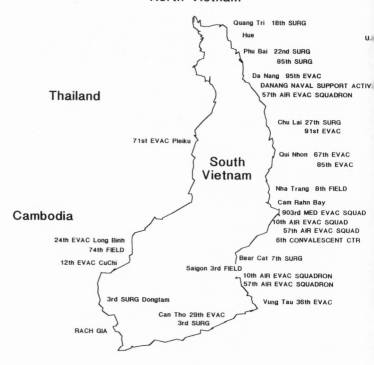

North Vietnam

Thailand

Cambodia

South
Vietnam

Quang Tri 18th SURG
Hue
U.
Phu Bai 22nd SURG
85th SURG

Da Nang 95th EVAC
DANANG NAVAL SUPPORT ACTIV
57th AIR EVAC SQUADRON

Chu Lai 27th SURG
91st EVAC

71st EVAC Pleiku

Qui Nhon 67th EVAC
85th EVAC

Nha Trang 8th FIELD

Cam Rahn Bay
903rd MED EVAC SQUAD
10th AIR EVAC SQUAD
57th AIR EVAC SQUAD
6th CONVALESCENT CTR

24th EVAC Long Binh
74th FIELD

12th EVAC CuChi

Bear Cat 7th SURG

Saigon 3rd FIELD
10th AIR EVAC SQUADRON
57th AIR EVAC SQUADRON

3rd SURG Dongtam

Can Tho 29th EVAC
3rd SURG

Vung Tau 36th EVAC

RACH GIA

Women

at War

The Story of Fifty Military

Nurses Who Served in Vietnam

ELIZABETH M. NORMAN

University of Pennsylvania Press
Philadelphia

STUDIES IN HEALTH, ILLNESS, AND CAREGIVING
Joan E. Lynaugh, Series Editor

A complete list of books in the series is available from the publisher.

All photographs used by permission.

10 9 8 7 6

Published by
University of Pennsylvania Press
Philadelphia, Pennsylvania 19104-4011

Library of Congress Cataloging-in-Publication Data

Norman, Elizabeth M.
    Women at war : the story of fifty miltary nurses who served in
Vietnam / Elizabeth M. Norman.
    p.   cm.
    Outgrowth of author's doctoral dissertation
    Includes bibliographical references (p.).
    ISBN 0-8122-8249-3. — ISBN 0-8122-1317-3 (pbk.)
1. Vietnamese Conflict, 1961–1975—Women—United States.
2. Vietnamese Conflict, 1961–1975—Medical care. 3. Nurses—United
States. 4. Nurses—Vietnam. I. Title.
DS559.8.W6N67   1990
959.704'37'0922—dc20   90-34487
[B]   CIP

**To Michael,
Joshua, Benjamin**

John and Dorothy

Contents

Acknowledgments

The process of locating military nurses who served in the Vietnam War was greatly expedited by Joan Barron, R.N. Her suggestions and contacts were useful in starting the study. Another nurse, Comdr. Cassie Greeley, USNR, NC, provided insightful comments on the questions I developed for the interviews.

Brig. Gen. Sarah P. Wells, USAF, NC (Ret.) helped me locate photographs to use in the book. Other nurses shared their war photographs: Capt. Mary Ann Gallagher Ibach, USNR, NC; Col. Sharon La France, USAFR, NC; Lt. Col. Mary Jo Rice, USAR, NC; Maj. Marra Peche, USAR, NC; former lieutenant Nancy Spears, USA, NC; former lieutenant Janice Stewart, USA, NC, and former lieutenant Martha Mosley, USA, NC. Thank you for your time and assistance.

Several nurses reviewed and reacted to my ideas presented in this book: Adm. Frances Shea Buckley, USN, NC (Ret.); Col. Sharon La France USAFR, NC; Brig. Gen. Diann A. Hale, USAF, NC (Ret.); Brig. Gen. Sarah P. Wells, USAF, NC (Ret.); former lieutenant Joan Furey, USA, NC and former captain Sara McVicker, USA, NC. Their detailed suggestions proved accurate and very useful.

My husband Michael edited the manuscript and helped me clarify themes and images in the book. For this, and everything else, thank you.

I also want to express my appreciation to the members of the New York University faculty who advised me through the dissertation process: Dr. Margret S. Wolf and Dr. Patricia Winstead-Fry. I am grateful to Dr. Joseph B. Giacquinta, who guided me in implementing research techniques I used. His willingness to share his knowledge and his commitment to students will serve as standards for me to follow in my academic career.

Many of my colleagues at Rutgers University were involved in various aspects of this book: Dr. Dorothy DeMaio, Dr. Noreen Mahon, Dr. Adela Yarcheski, Dr. Elsie Gulick, Mr. Mark Papianni, and Ms. Kim Morissey; thank you for your support.

Encouragement from my parents John and Dorothy Dempsey—both war veterans—has always given me a special edge.

Finally, I am indebted to the fifty women I interviewed in this study. Your stories and memories will be with me always.

Introduction

This book grew out of the rigors of the academic process—in short, it picks up where my doctoral dissertation ends. Seven years ago, I became interested in the military nurses who served in Vietnam. I was doing some summer reading—a popular book about Vietnam. In it, there were two accounts of nurses who had served in the war. It had never occurred to me, a nurse, that there had been women in the war. I was intrigued. That fall, as part of my work toward my Ph.D., I was assigned to write a paper for a nursing course that was taught by a professor who was particularly interested in history. The story of those two nurses had stayed with me, and I decided to use my academic assignment to learn more about the women who served as nurses in Vietnam. I discovered that virtually no one had been interested enough in the subject to pursue it. I found no statistics, no articles, just a two-page summary written by the army surgeon general in 1973. The academic in me was surprised: this seemed like such an obvious subject for study and exploration. The woman in me was alarmed: here was a part of history—the history of women—that might be lost. Who were these women? Why hadn't anyone written about them? What was it like to be a nurse in a war zone?

I decided to make the subject my dissertation. I wasn't committed to my subject, wasn't involved with it is any personal or political way. I had no particular view or message to send; rather, the idea of studying nurses who served in Vietnam simply seemed worthy.

I enjoyed the work during those early stages of research and I learned much about these women. But the more absorbed I became in the study, the more I came to realize that as I looked more closely at them, I was uncovering something of myself. My mother had been in the SPAR (the women's branch of the Coast Guard) during World War II. She spoke often of this time as being the best years of her life. She showed the family pictures of herself in a fitted blue uniform. She looked so young, so different from the woman who raised five daughters and worked full-time as a schoolteacher. I thought I might see in the women of Vietnam something of my mother and something of her generation. So it was to be a personal as well as a professional "project," a dissertation and a discovery.

When I began my work in 1983, the national indifference over the Vietnam war was just beginning to end. That year, the delayed celebration of the Vietnam veteran began. Parades, memorials, and written tributes appeared. Along with their male counterparts, nurses who served in Vietnam began to be seen in books and on television talk shows. But the public unveiling of these women was charged with controversy. A schism developed in their ranks. Some said the war was a good experience, some a bad one. Some claimed psychological scars, some said they had come home untouched. Everyone, it seemed, had a point of view she wanted to stress.[1]

The interviews I conducted for this book taught me that there was no standard experience or common reaction to the war. Rather, these fifty stories illustrate the variety and the incredible extremes of war. I thought it was important to show the spectrum of their experiences, that it was not one woman's story that was important, but all their stories, *together*.

The history of nursing is filled with accounts of Florence Nightingale, the first modern nurse and first scientific healer in our profession, and other early leaders. But the thousands of women who carry the profession forward every day in hospital unit in Vietnam. In all, they represent the span of the nursing experience in the armed forces in Vietnam. A more detailed description of the fifty women is the appendices of this book.

I chose to exclude civilian nurses, male nurses in the military, and those professionals who worked with war casualties in Thailand, Japan, Guam, Okinawa, and the Philippines. I wanted to keep the study focused on Vietnam, women, and the military. In no way did I mean to devalue these other nurses' service. Their contributions and experiences remain unexplored, and each group is worthy of its own study.

Only two of the women contacted refused to be interviewed. One said the memories were too painful; the other said she did not remember the details.

The rest could not have been more forthcoming. They welcomed me into their homes and onto their bases. The nurses in the military worked at the Pentagon, Bethesda Naval Hospital, McGuire Air Force Base in New Jersey. They would appear in their military uniforms—ribbons and rank smartly displayed. They would order subordinates to give us privacy and then lead me into some quiet place. Once the door was closed, the "officer," the military leader, was often left outside. Some stumbled through their stories. Some wept.

Those at home prepared coffee, offered cakes. A few would take the telephone off the hook and dig out their photo albums of the war.

Often, it seemed they could account for almost every day of their year-long tour in Vietnam. They could draw a map of their own hospital and list all the people and some of the patients who were there at certain times. "If I close my eyes, I can still smell the operating room, the ship's orders, and the patients," said a navy nurse who had worked on a hospital ship in 1966.

The interviews always followed the same pattern. We began with introductions and exchanged information about ourselves. I was usually asked if I was a veteran, what had brought me to the subject, and who I had interviewed. Sometimes, my subjects began to drift: they would sit back and begin to stare into space. When the interview ended they'd say, "I haven't thought about those things in years, but everything just kept flooding back to me."

Their stories became a chorus. During the last of the fifty interviews, I could not keep myself from crying with them. It was not my war. They were not my memories. But, listening to their stories of endless casualties, the bloody brutality of war, I began to get a sense of the loss and grief they carried. Their stories made the war real for me. Perhaps they will make it real for you as well.

1
Volunteering for the Vietnam War

Why would a woman choose to go to war—especially the war in Vietnam? Men did not line up at the recruiting stations and women did not gather under the sign of the Red Cross. We remember men as draft resisters and women as draft counselors. And yet, as figures from the Department of Defense show, the great majority of those who served in Vietnam—men and women—volunteered.[1] They did not shout about their choices. They went quietly. The fifty women in this book all volunteered for military service. Some joined the military to begin a career, some to get more training, some to pay for a nursing education. Thirty-four of the fifty volunteered to go to Vietnam. Only four of the others objected to being sent.

History and heredity made them go. Most nurses in the 1960s and early 1970s (the time of nurses' involvement in the war) were white, working class and middle class Catholic and Protestant daughters whose fathers were veterans of World War II and whose grandfathers recalled the Great War. Some were inspired by heroes like the fictitious Cherry Ames, the young nurse who bravely served her country in World War II and whose exploits were told in a series of popular books published in the 1940s and 1950s.[2] She was an inspiration, the female equivalent of John Wayne or Audie Murphy.

Going to war also was part of the adult American experience. There were war movies at Saturday matinees, large Memorial Day parades down Main Street, and a president who was a war hero. An army nurse who grew up in North Dakota remembered this patriotic atmosphere and had volunteered to go to Vietnam to show people, "A little town girl can serve her country and be a hero."

There were strong feelings of loyalty to country among the nurses. They had a sense of pride and a sense of duty. These women knew they could not be drafted like their brothers and high school friends, but they felt an equal responsibility to serve. "How could I say, 'Oh no, not me,' when men my age were going?" recalled another army nurse, "I really felt, 'How come not me?'" The result of this enthusiasm was an excess of nurses volunteering for Vietnam duty. In 1965, for example, navy leaders planned to commission the first hospital ship for service in the waters off Vietnam. Twenty-nine nurses were to be part of the first crew. Navy administrators quickly had a list of 400 nurses who requested duty on the ship, out of a total of 1,874 active duty nurses in the entire navy.[3]

Early in their lives, young girls learned the responsibilities of caring for others. While boys were outdoors playing baseball, girls were indoors playing house. Girls learned to view themselves in relation to others, as mothers, sisters, and friends—not as individuals.

As they grew up, nursing became a logical career choice. The task of caring for others is the core of the profession. And the war was an opportunity to care for others who really needed it—men their own age who were far from home, orphaned children, and wounded civilians. This was the profession at its most basic. No big medical bureaucracy, no stringent rules, just an opportunity to fulfill the basic, traditional female roles; to care and to feel needed. One nurse summed up the thoughts of others when she said, "Politics had nothing to do with it. I was very naive. But, if our men were fighting and dying, someone ought to be there taking care of them. We had to be there as nurses."

The antiwar movement, so prevalent on college campuses during the war, was missing from the hospital schools of nursing. During the 1960s, diploma schools—the term used to define hospital schools of nursing where the nurses received diplomas at the completion of three years of school—were the primary institutions for training nurses.[4] A woman spent those three years living in a dormitory, usually on the hospital grounds, and working long shifts on the hospital wards. Her education involved classes in anatomy, nutrition, and other sciences, and hospital practice. At the end of the third year, she graduated and prepared to take the registered nurse licensing examination. It was a cloistered, carefully monitored world. There was little time for or interest in questioning government policy. Not one of the fifty nurses in this study mentioned trying to avoid duty in Vietnam because of moral or political motives.

Not every nurse, however, went to Vietnam because of patriotism or loyalty to others. Just as men have long done, some nurses realized the personal benefits of going to a war zone. Here were the reasons this group of nurses volunteered for wartime duty:

Protective parents were left behind—"My father tore up my application to the Peace Corps so I joined the navy," said a woman who grew up in a strict Catholic household.

Another woman wanted to avoid a stifling future. "Everyone else in nursing school was going home to get married. I was not going to do that. I did not want to come home to Somerville, New Jersey, because I was afraid that in 35 years I would still be there."

A former army nurse said wartime duty was a chance for an adventure—"On a whim, my friend and I put in our papers to go to Vietnam. That's about all the thought I gave it!"

Going to Vietnam provided one nurse with a chance to travel to the exotic—"I always wanted to see the Orient and get out of Florida!"

Still another sensed work in an evacuation hospital would be a chance to test herself—"I wanted to see if I could do it. The patients on my ward who were recuperating from war wounds got my curiosity up. I also thought this is my generation's war. There would not be another chance again."

And for the career officer, the war was a chance to move up

the military ladder—"I was due to go overseas for my next [military] tour and the best opportunity for promotion was in Vietnam."

Regardless of the reason for volunteering, a few women gave deep thought into what the experience would really be like for them. It was a time in their lives when decisions were quick and consequences not pondered.

In 1956, the army instituted a Student Nurse Program to increase the number of nurses in uniform.[5] This program paid for the final years of nursing education in return for service after graduation. Twenty of the fifty women interviewed were in this program. These nurses entered the military at age twenty or twenty-one and most planned to stay only long enough to pay off their debt. The army was a good beginning for a professional nursing career. A few realized they might receive orders for Vietnam, but for most of these women the war seemed an improbable place. Most volunteered to go, but some were very surprised when they opened the manila order envelope.

In an effort to offset their fears, a few women in this study used a "buddy system" to go to Vietnam. Five army and navy nurses said this system permitted two friends who volunteered for wartime duty to serve at the same medical facility in Vietnam. They thought the presence of a friend might help them adjust to the long and difficult working hours and to the world of bunkers, air raid sirens, jungle heat, and typhoons.

Four of the nurses interviewed who were in the student nurse program did not volunteer for duty in Vietnam and did not want to go. These nurses had assumed that their mandatory service would be in the United States, Germany, or Japan. Their reluctance to go to Vietnam was more the result of professional insecurity—one women graduated from college in June and landed in Vietnam in November—and a lack of interest in the military as a lifelong career than any moral or political objection to the war. In the end, all four nurses followed orders and reported to Vietnam.

Parents were used to sending their sons off to war but not their daughters. Fathers frequently shared a sense of duty and expressed pride at their girls' decisions. At the same time, however, they worried about what would happen to their daughters' morals. Many fathers had served in World War II. They held strongly to the stereotype that only women of low moral character went into the military.[6]

Most nurses did not need their parents' permission to enter the military. They were at least twenty years old, considered adult and able to sign the necessary papers. Fathers worried about morality, but daughters wanted the military life and the war held sway. In the end one father, a career army officer, realizing the decision had been made, passed on an old military tradition to his daughter. "Do not," he said, as she went out the door for basic training, "volunteer for anything."

Mothers also could feel pride, but most nurses remember the tears and the upset that greeted their decisions. These mothers had guided their daughters through school and Girl Scouts and puberty. Their daughters had even chosen a good female profession. Going into the military and going to Vietnam did not fit the picture. There was too much that was unknown.

When the nurses volunteered for the war, the current feminist movement was just beginning. The concept of the "dependent daughter" who relied on her parents for emotional support and guidance was the norm.[7] Parents were protective. The thought of their daughter going to a war zone was both unnerving and frightening. There were no guidelines, no rules, and no precedents for parents to follow. Once she was in Vietnam, there was no way to protect her from danger, strain, loneliness, and men. One nurse summed up a typical parental reaction: "My parents were very upset and they said they did not understand me. My older brother had not even been to Vietnam. And here I was, their only daughter, going off to war."

Military leaders did not prepare nurses for Vietnam with the same rigor as for the men. Formal professional training took place in nursing school or at civilian and military hospitals. The amount of professional experience the nurses had before going to Vietnam varied greatly—from those with less than six months of work as a nurse to women with fifteen or twenty years of work experience in operating rooms, emergency rooms, and hospital units. Generally, the more professional nursing experience prior to Vietnam, the more confident the nurse.

Most older, experienced nurses were operating room nurses

who were in great demand during the Tet Offensive of 1968. One woman, an experienced circulating and scrub nurse in the operating room, received twenty-four hours' notice in February 1968 to report for duty in Vietnam. She received her orders on Friday and on Saturday was on an airplane heading for Da Nang, South Vietnam. There was little time to train nurses in the complex procedures used in operating rooms filled with traumatic war injuries from large scale military offensives. Experienced nurses relied on years of work in civilian and military hospitals to meet the demands of twenty-hour days around operating tables.

Nine women in this study had more than five years of professional experience when they went to Vietnam. They brought to the war a varied background particularly suited for wartime work. Two of them were veterans of the Korean War. When asked if there were differences between the Korean and Vietnam wars, one nurse said, "In Vietnam, there was no front, the war was all around us. We were always in danger of attack. And the casualties were worse. The helicopters would bring in severely wounded boys who would have died on the battlefield in another war. And the nurses took so much of it to heart." Experience and maturity helped this group of nurses face the timeless as well as the unique aspects of Vietnam.

Another nurse had spent three years on the Project Hope hospital ship caring for people in South America and West Africa. The poverty and foreign culture in Saigon was not a shock to her. Rather, working in the Vietnam War as an air force flight nurse presented the challenge she wanted after her Third World experience.

Personal backgrounds helped prepare some young women for Vietnam service. The nurses who grew up on farms in the Midwest and in Pennsylvania were used to living without amenities. Sharing quarters in Quonset huts or tents or simple buildings on a military compound recalled the camping or farmhouse rooms of their rural childhood. Similarly, those women who grew up in military families and moved around the world as children felt they had the flexibility to adjust to the very different living situations in Vietnam.

One young woman was more prepared than others for the tragedy she would see in the war. She followed her military orders knowing there was more than adventure and professional challenge in wartime work. Her husband had died in combat two months before she left to serve in an army evacuation hospital. His death did not make her afraid to go to Vietnam. It sobered her. She knew this was a place where, she said, "one could get killed."

Formal preparation varied between the services. The army offered an eight to ten week preparation course at Fort Sam Houston in Texas. The navy had no specific training program but required nurses to serve at least one two-year tour before going overseas. This minimum requirement insured that all nurses would have some professional experience and skills before working on the hospital ships or at naval hospitals in Vietnam. Air force nurses attended a standard two-month flight school where they received in-flight training. The first weeks in Vietnam were spent with an instructor who supervised them as they worked in different types of aircraft and prepared patients for evacuation flights.[8]

Endurance training or information about the health beliefs and practices of the Vietnamese were not part of this preparation. It was as if government planners believed nurses were going to "just nurse" rather than to spend a year working long hours with a very different people and, at times, witnessing and participating in the dangers of war.

Despite any professional or personal experience that helped prepare them for Vietnam, most of the fifty nurses agreed that nothing could ever adequately help an individual face the reality of war. A former army nurse echoed the feelings of others: "In retrospect, there is no way, even if I had served three tours of duty [three years], that I could have been ready for Vietnam. It's the human factor. It's the inability to conceive that this [war] really can happen."

One woman shared the information she received from the Department of the Army before leaving for the war. The packet included a map of South Vietnam showing the major cities and military commands; a letter from the deputy commanding general of the army; and guidelines for arrival, personal conduct, security, clothing, personal finances, savings programs, currency control, billets and mess, privately owned firearms, baggage, army facilities, time zones, duty hours, educational facilities, armed forces radio and television, R and R program and leave, and legal matters.

There were additional guidelines for army nurse corps officers regarding uniforms, library services, mail service, post exchanges, curfew, and off-limits policy, and a list titled, "Do's and Don'ts in South Vietnam":

DO be courteous, respectful and friendly!
DON'T be overly familiar with the Vietnamese.

DO learn and respect Vietnamese customs;
DON'T forget that you are a foreigner in this country.

DO be patient with the Vietnamese attitude toward time;
DON'T expect absolute punctuality.

DO appreciate what the South Vietnamese have endured;
DON'T give the impression that the US is running the war.

DO learn some useful Vietnamese phrases;
DON'T expect all Vietnamese to understand English.

DO be helpful when you can;
DON'T insist on the Vietnamese doing things your way.

DO learn what the South Vietnamese have to teach;
DON'T think Americans know everything.

At the beginning of the packet was a letter from the Chief Nurse USARV (United States Army Republic Vietnam)

23 May 1969

Dear Lieutenant:

It is indeed a pleasure to welcome you to Vietnam. I know you are looking forward to this assignment and will find it challenging, interesting and most rewarding.

It is recommended that all the personal items you will need to begin duty, be hand-carried by you to Vietnam. Hold baggage takes 2–3 months to arrive, therefore, you must bring your mandatory clothing items in your personal baggage.

Bear in mind weight restrictions on luggage and select items to bring accordingly. Please identify all luggage that you bring and mark personal items and clothing with name or other identification.

The green cord uniform is authorized to travel to Vietnam. Bring 2 sets of white duty uniforms, leaving the remaining sets available for subsequent mailing in the event they are required at a later date. Civilian dress is desired for off-duty wear.

All incoming flights are met by representatives from the USARV Transient Detachment to assist you. You will be directed at a specific time for a personel [sic] interview with me for assignment instructions and orientation.

Enjoy your leave, have a nice trip over and best wishes in your new assignment. We look forward to having you.

Sincerely,
Nellie L. Henley
LTC, ANC
Chief Nurse, USARV

2
Arriving in Vietnam

The twenty-four-hour flight to Vietnam was more than an endurance test of cramped legs, unappetizing food, and a sleepless night. It was, for many, the first time they thought of danger and death. Boisterous passengers, especially those men returning for a second tour in the war, suddenly became quiet when the coast of Vietnam came into view. A few soldiers began to put together their M-16 rifles. For the nurse, often the only female officer on board the aircraft, the last hour in the air was a time when fear began to mingle with the curiosity she had felt during preparations for her year-long tour. There was fear for her own safety and fear that many of the men who sat around her would never see home again. The daily and weekly casualty figures she had heard on nightly television newscasts took on a new, personal meaning. The Vietnam War was now part of the nurse's consciousness.

For six of the nurses, there was little time to ponder these thoughts. The aircraft or the airport where they would land was under enemy fire. The war was immediate and frightening. One nurse recalled ''We were not far off the coast [of Vietnam] when the captain announced they [the enemy] were mortaring the airfield. He said he was going to drop us off and get right back into the air. The plane made a steep landing into the airfield. They opened the door. We ran out and the troops going home ran on the plane. We were told to follow the person in front of us into a bunker. Unfortunately, I had high heels on. Did you every try to run in them?'' She laughed at the memory of herself in fashionable shoes trying to keep up with men running in combat boots.

Military men arrived in Vietnam in their working fatigue uniforms. Nurses arrived in their dress uniforms: a two-piece suit, hat, high-heeled shoes, gloves, and a pocketbook. Nurses were supposed to look neat, feminine, and professional even in the middle of a war. These uniforms proved dangerous for some nurses; others merely found them difficult to wear while climbing up a hospital ship's gangway or felt self-conscious at the curiosity they caused. People quickly noticed American women among the men in combat green.

As the new, inexperienced military personnel mingled with returning weary veterans in the suffocating tropical heat, the sights, sounds, and smells of a very poor, different world became apparent. Who was the enemy? Everyone dressed the same and looked so poor. In an era before terrorist bombings became commonplace, the sight of buses with anti-grenade screens and jeeps with mounted machine guns escorting arriving troops was unnerving. Nurses could no longer avoid being part of the excitement and the risk.

Before leaving the United States, the navy and air force nurses in this study knew their assignments. These women went directly to hospitals or hospital ships or air evacuation squadrons in Vietnam. The navy nurses worked on two hospital ships, the USS *Repose* and the USS *Sanctuary*—or at Naval Support Activity (NSA) Da Nang Hospital. One navy nurse worked as an adviser to the Vietnamese at Rach Gia, a French provincial hospital. The air force nurses in this study either were stationed in Vietnam and flew air evacuation missions from base to base or flew to Vietnam from the Philippines to pick up casualties and transport them to Japan and the United States.

After arriving in the war zone, Army Nurse Corp officers, who made up the largest contingent of professional nurses in the Vietnam war, went to Long Binh, a huge American base west of

Saigon that served as the nurses' replacement depot.[1] There they were given a choice of assignments: field and convalescent hospitals that were large hospitals much like those in the United States; evacuation hospitals that had several hundred surgical and medical beds where most patients quickly moved through the system on their way home; and surgical hospitals which were smaller and where trauma surgery was performed. One army nurse in this study set up and worked at one of the two prisoner-of-war hospitals in Vietnam.

Early recollections of those first days illustrate the naivete of people new to war. One nurse was eating lunch on her first day in Cu Chi, an army base near the Cambodian border. A siren went off. She thought it signaled an air raid, started to move, but noticed everyone else continued to eat lunch. The noise was just the twelve o'clock whistle.

A Navy nurse recalled sitting in a boat ferrying personnel to the USS *Repose*. She looked up and saw people on the deck of a hospital ship yelling and clapping for her. She thought it was a nice way to make newcomers feel warm and welcome. Later she learned the clapping was not a welcome but rather applause, for a "new" person on board ships meant a "veteran" was going home. Everyone was happy to see replacement. After a few weeks on board ship, this nurse joined others on the deck "welcoming" new stateside personnel.

For others, the welcome was more somber. One navy commander, an operating room nurse with fifteen years of experience, reported for duty on board ship. The chief nurse told her to get some rest before starting work. She walked to the private quarters. Here, she learned there were only spaces for thirty women on the hospital ships. Until transfers and nurses going home left, the new replacements were homeless. She was sent to rest in the sick officers' quarters. (Segregating ill officers from enlisted troops maintained military protocol.) She entered the quarters and smelled an unfamiliar odor. The last people to use the room had been burn patients. The smell of burned skin and muscle is pungent and unique, like rancid barbecue. It permeates everything from the lining of one's nose to one's mattress. Before she fell off to sleep, she wondered what had happened to the burned men.

The standard tour of duty in Vietnam for all military person-nel was twelve months (U.S. Marines served thirteen-month tours). The initial three months in the war were a time to settle in and become accustomed to the routines and the people. Nurses tended to be very sociable and share stories about home. They sought out the people who would become their friends.

The women adjusted to cold showers, latrines, and small shared living quarters called "hooches" in the army and air force and "cabins" in the navy. It was also a time to watch and observe the veterans—those people who had been in Vietnam for six months or more. War-seasoned nurses helped newcomers learn necessary professional skills. For example, during a mass casu-alty situation, newcomers quickly learned how to prepare twenty wounded men for surgery in an hour. It did not take long to learn the special skills needed for wartime work. There were no trial-and-error situations and little time to practice. Motivation among the nurses was high to become proficient and responsible. The reason many nurses enlisted in the military—to provide quality care to wounded soldiers—remained strong. There also was a general understanding among the women that the more secure the nurse felt with her skills the easier the settling-in process.

In addition to these adjustments, army nurses noticed an unwritten rule of acceptance. Except for those nurses stationed in Saigon, where nurses wore the traditional white dress, battle fatigues were the standard uniform. There was a pecking order to the degree of fade in the fatigues. Bright green fatigues, fresh issue, meant the person was new to the war and was to be taken very lightly. Fatigues faded by many washings meant the wearer rated respect.

Chief nurses assigned the new replacements to specific wards: the emergency or receiving ward, intensive care unit, operating room, recovery room, neurologic unit, orthopedic unit, maxillofacial ward, postoperative unit, medical unit, Vietnamese unit. Air force nurses joined an air evacuation team.

Even in Vietnam, there was an average day. Nurses spent twelve hours a day, six days a week, caring for the sick and wounded. Alarm clocks were set for 6:00 A.M. People woke up to the playing of the "Star-Spangled Banner" over loudspeakers. There was an early morning camaraderie in the ward room or mess hall as people lined up for coffee. Then came work. Nurses collected samples for laboratory tests, dispensed medications, and changed bloody dressings. Flight nurses prepared patients for evacuation and monitored them as they flew from the battlefields to hospitals in Vietnam, Japan, Okinawa, the Philippines, or the United States. Fatigue was not a problem during these average seventy-two-hour weeks. The nurses were young and had stamina. Wartime nursing was the profession at its most basic. Life revolved around work.[2]

The sensitivity that some of the women had used to provide comfort to patients back home sometimes overwhelmed them in a world with badly injured and dying young men. Comforting words and touch had to take place quickly when so many young men needed so much care. Time took on a different meaning. One nurse felt she was caught up in an eddy, in a craziness she could not control. The nurses' age had little effect on their initial reactions to war injuries. For example, a woman in the study was in her late thirties when she went to Vietnam. She had worked in various positions for more than a decade prior to the war. Despite her extensive background, she found the casualties upsetting. She said, "I couldn't stand the wounds. I couldn't eat meat. I began to live on soups, peanut butter, eggs, and bread. Was there a purpose to all this? What a waste to see all those young kids [patients]."

The stories of the movie and book heroes suddenly seemed hollow. "I quickly learned," one nurse said, "That I was not in a John Wayne movie. The devastating injuries just came in and came in and I remember thinking, 'How is it possible for people to do this to each other?'" This surprise, however, soon turned to anger. Anger at the war, anger at the lost young lives. It was not until years later that these nurses came to diffuse their anger; they realized then the Vietnam War was no different from every other war. No one individual could control the outcome. They now understood that young lives inevitably were going to be lost.

The typical soldier who arrived for treatment had many different types of injuries. It was unusual to see a single gunshot wound. More likely, nurses would work on someone who suffered from multiple traumatic injuries. For example, a navy nurse remembered one patient who had stepped on a land mine and lost both legs. The impact of the blast perforated his ear-drums. He also fractured both arms when he hit the ground.

Shrapnel, the tiny metal fragments released from exploding devices, could penetrate areas not seen by a doctor or nurse. If undetected, shrapnel fragments would become infected. To prevent this complication, all preoperative patients were sent to X-ray for pictures of their entire body. Surgeons then examined the X-rays to locate and later remove any hidden metal.

Operating rooms became crowded with two or three surgical teams working on the same patient. One team would repair leg damage while another team worked to close up abdominal trauma. Most wounds were contaminated with dirt and easily became infected. Surgeons would not close up amputations or gunshot wounds in the operating rooms. Infected wounds left open healed better. At a later time, surgeons in Japan or in stateside hospitals closed these wounds.

Nurses also found themselves in wards filled with patients diagnosed with tropical diseases like malaria, cholera, even snake and monkey bites. There were the exotic diseases of bubonic plague and tetanus, usually found only in nursing textbooks. Caring for people with medical disease was beneficial to these women for two reasons: one, it provided a change from combat trauma, and two, it was an opportunity to see and to work with "illnesses" many others in their profession would never see.

There were opportunities to break the everyday routine and leave the confinement of the hospitals. As a humanitarian gesture, military leaders established Medical Civilian Action Patrols (called Medcaps) to bring American health care to civilians.[3] Twenty of the fifty nurses in this study went on these missions. They were sent, for example, to civilian hospitals to work in the operating rooms; prisons to perform physical examinations; local schools to dispense medications; villages, to teach the inhabitants how to use soap and water and how to dress a war wound; dental clinics to help pull teeth from people who had never had dental work. One nurse helped set up a venereal disease clinic for the local prostitutes. Not all off-base time involved health care: one navy nurse taught English to students at a local high school in Da Nang.

The two most frequently mentioned Medcap destinations were orphanages and a leprosarium near the sixty-seventh Army Evacuation Hospital. One by-product of the war was the need for the many orphanages which were all over South Vietnam. These homes were magnets for nurses who could give and receive so much affection during their time spent with the children. After vaccinating and de-worming the children, nurses told nursery stories buried under a pile of four- and five-year-old orphans. They also distributed clothes their mothers collected at Sunday church services. It was hard not to return to the children week after week. The children provided a sense that normal life functions—like growing up—went on in spite of all the suffering around them.

Qui Nhon is a Vietnamese city that faces the South China Sea. French nuns, reminders of the earlier foreigners who fought in Vietnam, ran a leprosarium in this city. Leprosy is a communicable disease caused by *Mycobacterium leprae* bacteria. The disease can cause skin lesions, numbness in the hands and feet, muscle weakness, and paralysis.[4] It is a disease that dates from Biblical times, and is still found in poor, underdeveloped countries. Fingers and toes can fall off because of damage to small nerves and blood vessels. "Spontaneous amputation" is the medical term used to describe this disease's progression. Isolation of the leprosy patient in leprosariums is not necessary when specific antibiotics to kill are bacteria are administered but in the 1960s the physical and psychological stigma of leprosy remained strong. The nuns encouraged the army nurses to come to the leprosarium during their days off and work with a disease few other Americans knew even existed any more. They also provided another incentive to visit the leprosarium: after the nurses worked in surgery or performed dressing changes on the patients, the nuns served a magnificent French lunch and allowed the nurses to use their private beach facing the South China Sea. A day at the leprosarium was a chance to step back from the war, a chance to enjoy the beauty of the Vietnamese sea coast, and a chance to meet religious missionaries.

By the time nurses had served in Vietnam for three to six months—the middle of their wartime tours—their worlds had reversed. The war was home and stateside was far away. Nurses felt comfortable with the people around them. They had their circle of trusted friends and workers. Family events and news were known only through letters and "care" packages of food. The United States seemed a distant past and distant future.

The pace of life was directly related to the flow of casualties and helicopters dictated an incredibly busy or slow day in the hospitals. After three months in Vietnam, hospital personnel could listen and identify by sound alone the type of helicopter approaching the flight pad and whether it was empty or full of casualties. At the sound of a full helicopter everyone reported to work—from the officers' club, the mess hall, and the living quarters. Everything, including work, went to extremes in Vietnam. Nurses worked either busy shifts where they never stopped or slow shifts that dragged on as supplies were checked and re-ordered. The war was a macabre parade of wounded patients, new friends, and arriving helicopters.

In Buddhist Vietnam the Christmas holiday took on a different image. The hot and rainy jungle replaced the cold and snow of home. Vietnamese soldiers and civilians watched and wondered at the strange behavior of the nurses. Why would they hang mistletoe in hospital doorways? Why decorate plaster leg casts with red and green pictures? Why set up cardboard fireplaces and green plastic trees in the wards? This blend of culture and religion was as strange to the Vietnamese as the Buddhist Tet holiday was to the American military.

Christmas was a social time at the military bases and on the ships. Two icons of American life came to Vietnam for the holidays. The first was a Sears Roebuck catalog, the source book for the decorations and trinkets so foreign to the Vietnamese. It took an average of two weeks to deliver an order from this company to the nurses' quarters in Qui Nhon or Pleiku. Unwrapping the Sears package and examining the familiar contents was cause for a party and a break in the work monotony. Home seemed as far away as a Sears order form.

The second Christmas icon was Bob Hope. Nurses scrambled to attend his annual shows of jokes, songs, dances, and "cheesecake." These women treasure pictures of themselves seated in the front of an audience of thousands of GIs. The nurses are hard to see in the pictures because they dressed in the same hat and uniform as the men. They are a glaring contrast to the actresses and beauty queens on stage in slinky gowns and short dresses. Some women are sitting on the ground, legs crossed, laughing at the man with a golf club on the stage. Other women are standing next to patients on stretchers who have intravenous fluid running into their veins. Attending Bob Hope's show was a chance to take part in a holiday military tradition that began in their fathers' war two decades earlier.

Christmas was a time to be with friends and patients. Nurses dressed as Santa Claus and sang carols throughout the hospitals. At midnight on December 24, 1967, a voice came over the loud-speaker on the USS *Repose* to announce flight quarters for a sleigh and eight tiny reindeer. Not all Christmases were happy, of course. Nurses at an army evacuation hospital forgot Christmas when 28 wounded Americans arrived for treatment on Christmas Eve. It seems South Vietnamese soldiers had miscalculated coordinates; mortars and artillery landed on top on American soldiers by mistake. Starting blood transfusions and dressing head wounds replaced gifts and turkey dinner that year.

After six months in Vietnam, nurses and other military personnel could leave the war zone for a short period of "R and R"—rest and relaxation leave. Nurses headed to Hong Kong, Taiwan, Australia, Bangkok, Tokyo, and the Philippines for a five day vacation. They planned to shop, eat in restaurants, sleep in soft beds, and lounge on the beaches. Arriving in these vacation cities, some women recognized how much they had changed. "I was scared when I landed," said one nurse who went to Hong Kong, "because it was so open and there was so much activity. Then I realized I had been in a very strange environment and this was the real world. I couldn't get enough of it."

Another nurse remembers walking down a busy city street in Sydney, Australia, when a construction worker started up a jack-hammer. Using a reflex she had developed during mortar attacks in Da Nang, she dove into the first storefront opening she saw. She realized she was in a jewelry store and bought a ring to cover up her embarrassment. Sixteen years later, she was wearing this ring during the research interview.

When they returned to Vietnam from R and R, the nurses held no illusions about the war as they boarded planes to return to their military assignments. As the aircraft lifted off and headed toward the war, these women knew exactly what they were returning to do.

3

The Professional Strains and Moral Dilemmas of Nursing in Vietnam

There is a timelessness to a nurse's recollections of war. Whether she served near the trenches of France in World War I, in North Africa during World War II, or in Cu Chi, South Vietnam, each remembers long hours working with grievously injured men. The recollections that follow in many ways correspond to Vera Brittain's *Testament of Youth,* her account of World War I nursing, or Theresa Archard's *G.I. Nightingale,* a record of nurses in the North African and Italian campaigns of World War II.

Wartime nursing is particularly stressful because of the age and the severity of injury seen in the patients. It is easier to accept disability, even death, in the elderly than in the young. An elderly person has experienced work, friends and family, sports and good books, health and illness, seasons and holidays. A young person is only on the verge of such a life. Most patients in Vietnam were so young that nurses often looked at them to see if the boys lying on the stretchers or beds were high school classmates. More likely, wounded soldiers reminded the nurses of their younger brothers or friends. In Vietnam, the average age of the nurses interviewed was twenty-two years, the average age of enlisted men was nineteen years.[1]

The rapid evacuation system for the wounded saved many lives that would have been lost in previous wars. Casualties from the battlefield could arrive at hospital receiving wards (emergency rooms) within minutes of injury. For example, one woman remembered looking at the wristwatch on a patient as she prepared him for surgery. His watch had stopped seventeen minutes earlier, the moment he was wounded.

Mortality rates at military medical facilities were under three percent.[2] Although it salvaged lives, this system also created a dilemma about the quality of life left for some of the men. Nurses spoke of the guilt and confusion they felt when they sent severely disabled patients home. "Imagine," said one women, "working on a twenty-year-old soldier who only had one arm left. What did he have? I used to wonder what the rest of his life would be like. They were [all] in the prime of their lives." Every professional nurse sees death and trauma during the course of a career. Nurses who work in war zones deal with a lifetime of sadness and loss in one year.

The women felt maternal and protective instincts toward their young patients. These feelings often turned to anguish and anger when the nurses realized their patients would never be normal, functioning adults. It was emotionally wrenching for the nurses to look on row after row of comatose, brain damaged young soldiers. "I used to wonder," remembers one nurse, "if my patients had ever kissed or made love to a woman, if they graduated from high school or if they were in the middle of a college education. Did they have families of their own or were they planning to become fathers?"

Most questions remained unanswered. This lack of information had merit because once the nurses learned personal details, the objective lamina they had developed to shield themselves from emotional overload disappeared.[3] The pain and suffering belonged to people with names and personalities, not just patients.

A nurse who worked at the sixty-seventh Evacuation Hospital in Qui Nhon illustrated how difficult it was to uncover personal details about patients. One morning, she found a ditty bag next to her assigned patient. These bags were small canvas or leather carriers the men used to carry shaving equipment and other personal items. If a nurse had reason to go through a ditty bag, she usually found pictures of girl friends and wives, mothers and fathers, children and pets. This nurse opened her patient's bag to see if there was any useful information in it, for he could not talk to her. He had a severe head injury and burns. In his bag she found his ring from West Point Military Academy in New York. She looked at this young man, who was swathed in bandages because he did not have enough skin left to prevent bacteria from entering his body. It was hard for her to imagine him marching in the Long Gray Line with his sword and feathered hat at West Point's weekly dress parade. Suddenly, he became a person with an identity. It was harder to maintain a professional distance when the nurse knew her patient's home town and history.

The best way to deal with the emotion-charged hospital wards and planes was to concentrate on the physical work. Nurses could not sit and cry over these young men. Time was short. There was a fear that if one nurse started to cry the whole room would lose control because there was such sorrow. Sometimes, however, control was not possible. Something would break through the veneer. Whether it was a ditty bag, or hearing a young man whistle a tune through his bandages, or a simple request to listen to a story about a girl friend, a patient would remind a nurse that he was real. He was more than the diagnosis "gunshot wound to the chest."

Each nurse in this study was asked if there were any specific patients she remembered from Vietnam. Only one woman said she did not remember any of her charges. Fifteen years later, the other women, some in military uniform, others in professional dress or civilian clothes, cried as they remembered special patients. They spoke about many different young men who had moved them because of their youth, courage, and naiveté. Some women knew the names, ages, types of wounds, prognoses, even the sound of their patients' voices. Others simply recalled a look, a statement, or a gesture. The six stories that follow illustrate what it was like to work as a nurse in the emotionally intense atmosphere of war; they are examples of patients the nurses could not forget.

A young army lieutenant was working the night shift on an orthopedic ward at the large Third Field Hospital in Saigon. Her patients suffered from many different types of injuries: broken bones, crushed joints, torn ligaments, muscles, and nerves. These young men had been through their initial operations. They were in casts, dressings, and traction. As part of her job, the nurse helped her patients understand what had happened to them. Often, she would initiate the long process of recovery by encouraging these young men to write or call home. Some refused to worry their families. Others felt relief in hearing a familiar voice. Then there was one patient who reminded the nurse that, despite their energy, these were frightened young soldiers who faced enormous problems. She remembered, "One night a young boy was allowed to call home and speak to his parents. We wheeled his bed to the phone, which was in the middle of the ward. Here was this kid shouting into the phone in front of a room full of people. He was weeping and telling his parents he lost a leg. He cried and told them he would be all right."

While off duty, a navy nurse on board the USS *Repose* heard helicopters landing on the ship's deck. She was not startled or upset at the sound. It was 1968 and the pace of the war was fast. Marine corps casualties arrived at any time. All medical personnel tried to transfer patients quickly to hospitals in Guam, the Philippines, Okinawa, and Japan so that shipboard beds would be available for the newly wounded. So many patients came and went during the early months of 1968 that it was possible for the nurses to remain detached from the dozens of young marines who still wore short hair and sat up straight—even in wheelchairs. This nurse admired their enthusiasm, but one day she came to see that the famous Marine character was not enough:

New casualties were admitted during the night. I came on duty the next morning, and as I made rounds [checked patients] I saw this marine doing push-ups with his chest tube, urinary drainage bag, and IV [intravenous fluid] tube going into him. I wanted to laugh at his grit! The day before, he'd been wounded in the chest and abdomen. He spent the previous evening in surgery. Think about the kind of human spirit he had. It turned out his pancreas was involved and he eventually died. I often think about him and tell my [nursing] students about the heart he displayed.

Two years earlier on the same hospital ship, another navy lieutenant worked in the operating room. She usually saw her patients once and talked to them while surgical preparations were carried out. Occasionally a patient returned for more surgery—to remove dead skin, drain an infection; or amputate a limb the doctors had tried to save earlier. These last cases were particularly sad for this nurse because it seemed as though the mutilation should stop during or right after a battle. Each surgery made these men less whole and more disabled. One surgery was made even more poignant by the physique and reaction of the patient. She recalled: "a Marine already had one leg amputated. His other leg was going bad [losing blood circulation] and we were trying to save it. I was in the operating room when the surgeon told him he'd have to take off the other leg. This marine was a big, strapping guy. He said, 'Doc, you gotta do what you gotta do.'"

One air force nurse was adjusting to the long hours of flying patients from battlefields to hospitals throughout South Vietnam. Each day medics carried dozens of wounded soldiers through the aircraft doors on bloodied ponchos or litters. The first thing she did was to check the snugness of their dressings to make sure that no one hemorrhaged during the short flight. Her conscious patients reacted to their injuries with a variety of emotions. Some sobbed, but most lay quietly in the aircraft. She joked with them, held their hands, and gave them something to drink. One day, however, her humor left her: "As the plane lifted off, I pulled back the covers on this guy to see if he was bleeding. He had an AK [above the knee] amputation of the right leg. Between his left leg and the amputation was a Purple Heart. He reached down and picked it up. He was so proud of it. 'Isn't it neat?' he asked me, 'A general gave this to me.' I'm standing there looking at this kid and I wanted to cry."

Another navy lieutenant found it easy to identify those patients who were going to die. After a few weeks in Vietnam, she knew those patients arrived unconscious with gray-colored skin, glazed, unblinking eyes, and very shallow breathing. She never came to know these marines. Occasionally, a mortally wounded patient would not fit this description. All the sadness and loss in the war came through in these patients. She remembered one in particular.

A nineteen-year-old came in with abdominal wounds and an undetected hole in the back of his head. We'd pump blood into him and it would pour out the back. He was fully conscious. It was late at night. As I get him ready to go to the OR, he's talking to me saying, "My name is . . ."—thank God I don't remember it—"I'm from . . . I have a little sister . . . please . . . my parents." He knew he was going to die and he made me promise to write to his parents, which I did. Twenty minutes after he died, the song "Born Free" is played over the tape recorder. It was tough. It was tough.

A twenty-two-year-old lieutenant spent her entire year-long tour working in the intensive care unit with the most critically injured patients. She became practiced at soothing their fears and easing their pain. There were three patients she remembered from that year because they seemed to her to be possessed with a strength—or naiveté—beyond her grasp. She could do little for these three, but their cases still haunt her today. One of these patients was "a kid with three amputations. Only one leg was left. He went into the service right out of high school. He wanted to know if there was a Bible around. He asked me to please get him a Bible. His mother told him there were going to be days like this and he needed to read his Bible. My God."

What ever happened to these men? Once patients left the wards or aircraft, word of their recovery or fate rarely reached the nurses who had treated and come to know them. Thus these professional clinicians were not able to complete the most basic of cycles—a job started, a job finished. They did not, in short, have the satisfaction of knowing the outcome of their work.

Eighty-two percent of the nurses interviewed never found

out how their patients fared back in the United States. While most nurses wanted to know what happened to the patients, nine women preferred to remain uninformed. These women were content knowing the patients lived to get to the next phase of recovery. For the others, however, this lack of information fed the stress of their wartime tour.

Trained to care more for their comrades than for themselves, many of the wounded men displayed a selflessness that at first confused and unsettled the nurses. It was easier to comfort a person who cries out in pain—a predictable response—than someone who ignores an injury. An army lieutenant stationed at an evacuation hospital remembered the incident that taught her how upsetting such generosity could be. This nurse was the daughter of a career enlisted man and was very familiar with military behavior. It was not until Vietnam that she realized combat changed men used to protocol into fiercely devoted comrades.

She spoke about a night when dozens of casualties suddenly appeared in the receiving ward where she worked. A badly wounded army sergeant refused treatment from her until all the wounded men from his platoon received attention. He simply sat in the corner and never said a world while the nurses worked on his men. He embodied the unwritten slogan among the combat forces—"How's my buddy, take care of my buddy before me." People who were badly hurt were supposed to cry. People were supposed to be frightened. A normal reaction produces a normal response. Nurses can be caring and comforting to such patients. To watch this twenty-one-year-old sergeant waiting for treatment was a jittery experience. The army lieutenant did not relax until the sergeant was on his way to the operating room for overdue surgery.

Nurses in all three military branches witnessed selflessness in their patients. Air force nurses carried baloney sandwiches and milk on board the aircraft to feed the wounded men being ferried from battlefield to hospital. Before taking any of it, the men would always ask if there was enough food for everyone on board. Many of the wounded had been living in "the field"—in jungle foxholes and eating canned food—for months. The thought of fresh milk must have been enticing, but a friend's comfort came first. Nurses came to understand that the camaraderie combat soldiers developed living and fighting together carried over from the rice paddies to the medical evacuation planes and receiving wards.

But such personal indifference unnerved even experienced nurses who went to Vietnam confident in their ability to deal with suffering patients. For example, one navy nurse went to Vietnam with more than ten years of operating room experience. A young marine with a hand injury came to the operating room where she worked for surgery. He was not badly hurt but his story was horrifying. His unit had been surrounded by an enemy regiment and wiped out. He hid under his dead buddies for two days until a platoon rescued him. At night he heard the North Vietnamese mutilating his friends. After he arrived on the hospital ship, his only concern was to find out what had happened to his captain, whom he had seen shot. The navy nurse saw this captain and told the young marine that his captain was fine. "This kid reaches out," she said, and began to cry softly, "and thanks me for being so kind and good and taking care of him. I got out of his room and cried. All he'd been through and he's thanking me." Despite his ordeal, he had retained his humanity. His humanity was a vivid contrast to the elemental cruelty all around the nurses.

In this kind of world, the nurses felt they had to be as emotionally strong as their wounded patients. How, they asked themselves, could they complain about their work when these wounded men did not complain? The most common way in which the nurses reacted to the men's selflessness was to insulate themselves, to build up a shield that allowed them to work. Once the nurses lost their objectivity, it became difficult to work. Thus they kept hidden the most common and predictable of emotions—anger, sadness, sorrow, and pity. It was not until many years after the war that the women reexamined their wartime emotional repression. For example, twelve years after she returned home, one former army nurse spoke about reliving her wartime episodes. She let herself feel all the emotions she had buried in Vietnam. Finally, she was able to grieve for all the loss and sadness she had experienced in the war. "I feel much better,'' she said. She never will accept or fully understand what happened, but she does feel a sense of reconciliation.

When the sound of the helicopters was stronger and louder than usual, experienced nurses knew a mass casualty situation was about to occur. Large numbers, sometimes 150 patients in two hours, would arrive for treatment. Hospital personnel, even those off duty, left their living quarters, the officers' club, or the PX store and came to work. More than half of the nurses in this study (62 percent) remembered mass casualty situations when the work day expanded to twenty-four, thirty-six, or forty-eight continuous hours. Those nurses stationed in Vietnam during the 1968 Tet Offensive and Counteroffensive regularly experienced these situations. The timing of mass casualty situations was as unpredictable as the timing of the battles that caused them. For example, on Easter Sunday 1970, nurses at the Third Surgical Hospital in Dongtam began admitting soldiers wounded in a nearby battle in the dense jungle of the South Vietnamese Delta region. Three days later, the last wounded soldier from the battle was treated and the hospital team could finally rest. No one remembered the holiday.

Researchers have recently examined the statistics of the Naval Support Activity (NSA) Da Nang Hospital during the 1968 Tet Offensive. Their report illustrated how busy and efficient the medical and nursing care was at this medical facility:

- From January to June 1968, the death rate was 2.92 percent with 2,021 admissions.
- The greatest numbers of deaths were due to rifle/pistol injuries followed by artillery/rocket/mortar injuries.
- The average time a soldier spent in Vietnam before injury was 5.3 months.
- The average time from injury to admission was 2.8 hours for men who were salvageable.
- The time from admission to surgery was 1.9 hours for those men received alive.
- The average length of hospital stay in Vietnam was 4 days.
- The 2,021 admissions had 8,430 wounds. Extremity

wounds accounted for 68.2 percent of all recorded injuries. Extremity wounds had the highest incidence but lowest mortality rate. Penetrating wounds of the head, thorax, abdomen, or combination were found in 61 percent of all deaths.[4]

Mass casualty situations were startling.[5] Patient after patient arrived until litters holding soldiers covered the floor. Most soldiers had war wounds but some men arrived dehydrated, physically exhausted, or emotionally spent from the long hours in combat. There was barely room in the receiving wards to walk or work. Nurses stepped over litters with time only to watch patients' chests to see if they were breathing. They saw tubes and bodies and clothes and dirt. One nurse remembers cutting off pant leg after pant leg to expose wounds. Another remembered thinking, "Is there anybody left out there [fighting]?" When army hospitals became full, patients were evacuated to other facilities. At one point in 1968, the USS *Repose* was so overloaded with wounded surgical patients that men with medical problems like malaria were put on the ship's deck to recuperate.

Inexperienced nurses viewed these scenes and wondered where to begin work. Experienced personnel took control and initiated a familiar routine that they had used in previous situations.

The first step in the mass casualty process was a gruesome one. During the heat of battle, helicopters and air evacuation planes were enemy targets, so pilots would keep their engines running as litters and ponchos filled with bodies were thrown or put on board. Soldiers in the field did not have time to separate living and dead comrades. Air force nurses flying to hospitals, navy physicians and corpsmen on a ship's deck, and army physicians and medics on the helicopter pads outside the evacuation hospitals performed this task. One night, for example, there were sixty American bodies stacked on a ship's flight deck. Nurses avoided looking at this grim scene as they went to pick up the wounded.

"Triage" (French for sorting) was the next step in routine mass casualty care. Sick, wounded, or injured patients were classified with numbers to determine who would receive priority in treatment. Triage decisions were necessary for the efficient use of limited personnel, equipment, and facilities. The triage philosophy during mass casualty was "Salvage as many as you can."[6] This translated into allowing the least injured patients into the operating room first. Usually, the most experienced surgeon assumed overall responsibility for triage. It was the nurses' charge to decide in what order or priority patients would go into the operating rooms. Patients with head injuries might require six hours of valuable operating room time. Surgeons could operate on ten other patients during those six hours. So, the patients with head injuries went to the back of the line to wait their turn. Bobby (a pseudonym), a soldier from Texas with a head wound, was an example of someone who endured a triage decision. He was still alive after waiting through a whole night for his surgery. Bobby survived and went home but others died waiting.

The triage method seemed practical and necessary. How did nurses struggle with the decisions? Three nurses took a practical view. They concentrated on keeping some men alive and did not think about those who might die. The pace was fast and the judgments mechanical. Most of the nurses in the study, however, were unsettled by these difficult decisions. Saving lives is at the foundation of the profession. Letting a wounded person wait for treatment is anathema to nurses. The women found themselves going back to check on the worst patients in line. The method of treating the worst patient last is the opposite of the triage care practiced in the United States.[7] Ample personnel and operating rooms allow the most critically injured patient to gain top priority. But in Vietnam the nurses learned to adapt codes and skills to wartime demands.

There also was another type of triage practiced: an "Americans first" policy. The policy was unwritten, but everyone in the medical corps knew it. In the army and navy facilities, when operating rooms were busy, Vietnamese patients, especially known or suspected enemy agents and soldiers, waited until all the Americans were treated. In the air force, this policy meant that wounded Americans were never left behind on the battlefield. If aircraft were full of casualties, Vietnamese waited for the return flight. (Children, who were transported and worked on as quickly as possible, were the exception to this policy.)

Nurses rarely mentioned this policy for fear that people back home would not understand. In Vietnam, the nurses accepted it. Loyalty to other Americans was strong and the urge to save a wounded soldier overcame any reluctance to treat someone else first.

During triage work, physicians, corpsmen, and nurses found soldiers among the wounded who had no chance of survival; the unconscious men usually had severe head wounds. Corpsmen or medics put these soldiers in the corner of the receiving ward or intensive care unit behind screens to die. So many other patients needed immediate care, there was not time to help the hopeless. But these "expectant situations," as they were called, were professionally abhorrent to women who had a deep commitment to preserving life.

The task of monitoring expectant patients distressed everyone involved. In the busy ward atmosphere, nurse started blood transfusions, administered pain medications, explained surgical procedures, and pushed patients on gurneys to X-ray and to operating rooms. They worked on the survivors while behind the screen, a young man lay dying. After the neurosurgeon and chaplain left the "expectant" patients, it was the nurses' job to monitor the patients' vital signs until their hearts stopped beating. It was difficult to overcome the urge to "do something." All a nurse could do was touch and speak to these men. While listening for a heart-beat, a nurse would hold a man's hands and whisper into his ear. In Vietnam, and in other wars, women learned that nursing was more than healing. The women learned to measure death and soothe the way.

These expectant soldiers were strangers. Military "dog tags" were their only identification. The dog tags were two silver badges worn around a soldier's neck with his name, religion, military identification number, and blood type stamped on it. For the nurses, it was crucial that these anonymous soldiers not die alone or unattended. "When the end [death] was near," said a former army nurse who cried as she remembered these scenes, "I would just stand near them. I felt that his mother would feel better knowing that someone was standing with her son when he died." This timeless scene is one of sadness and loneliness. The soldier was every young man who went off to fight a war and never returned. The nurse was every women who mourned the wartime loss of a husband or son or brother.

When the mass casualties ended and the triage decisions had been made, hospital personnel paused. These people who had ignored their tiredness during the previous twenty-four to forty-eight hours yielded to their own fatigue. An army nurse who worked thirty-two hours in an intensive care unit while a nearby battle raged remembered "everyone just laying down and sleeping for the next two days."

Accompanying their fatigue was a sense of exhilaration. All nurses who took part in mass casualty situations shared this energizing and seemingly contradictory reaction. These women had been pushed to their personal limit and survived. They had met the challenge.

Morality provides individuals with general rules of conduct. We begin to learn moral behavior as children. Parents and other adults teach children not to cheat, steal, or hate others. Throughout life, moral judgments and behavior maintain a civilized society. Morality is what makes us human. Fighting a war, however, requires a change in these basic rules. The past moral history of an individual no longer corresponds with life in a war zone.

Military leaders condition soldiers to hate the enemy and act on this hatred by fighting to kill and win. The enemy takes on the image of evil, which makes them justified targets.[8]

Enlisted men learn this philosophy in basic training but all military personnel, including nurses, absorb this belief. In Vietnam, nurses were one with the larger military fraternity. They too were far from home and exposed to personal danger. Nurses worked grim and relentless days on the wards with wounded Americans. The North Vietnamese and Viet Cong were *the* enemy for nurses and fighting men.

The soldiers' attitude toward the Viet Cong and North Vietnamese was clear—kill or be killed. The nurses' feelings about the enemy were more clouded. Should known or suspected enemy soldiers receive the same nursing care as Americans?

In many hospitals, enemy soldiers were not segregated from the American wounded because of limited physical space. This environment compounded the nurses' moral dilemma regarding caring for the enemy. Nurses had a difficult time working on enemy soldiers at the same time that they could see wounded Americans lying in beds across the aisles. Some nurses felt angry and resentful.

For example, one day a nurse reported for duty at an intensive care unit and found Viet Cong saboteurs, American soldiers who were wounded in the saboteurs' attack, and civilians who happened to get caught in the crossfire lying side-by-side. This army nurse began her workday under the suspicious and resentful eyes of the American military police assigned to guard the enemy patients. The MPs were slow to help her and other nurses turn or lift enemy patients from their beds. The police were, however, quick to make disparaging remarks. "Why bother with this gook? [a derogatory term used for the Vietnamese]" they asked to the nurses. "Look what they did to these soldiers." The women did not answer them. "Your initial reaction," said the nurse who faced this group of patients and police, "was to strike the POWs. You are really angry at them because they hurt people you care about." Like most nurses in the study, she had volunteered for wartime duty for patriotic reasons. Helping the enemy recuperate and survive seemed disloyal.

One of the major differences between the Vietnam War and previous American wars was the wide-scale use of children, women, and older people as enemy saboteurs.[9] There was no front line in Vietnam. No one was sure who the enemy was, therefore everyone was suspect. It was easy to imagine the Vietnamese, especially the men, as enemies because they were a different race, a different culture. But, ten-year-old boys and young women—suspected terrorists—compounded the moral dilemma. The nurses did not easily view children and other women as evil enemies.

Nurses who reduced the enemy to objects found it was easy to deny their humanity. The enemy patients became patients who were not human. All subjective factors that distinguish one person from another were ignored. Nurses could then act on their hatred of the enemy by handling enemy patients roughly or by withholding or giving too little pain medication.

Two moral dilemmas, however, arose when nurses modified professional moral codes and embraced the military morality.

First, these morals violated a basic professional belief and attitude. Nursing is a moral art that places high value on the good of
the patient. Nurses accept the duty to care for all types of patients.[10] Promoting the health of the patients is more important
than military philosophy. The emotional consequence of know-
ingly hurting or providing substandard care was overwhelming
guilt. It was professionally impossible to be unfaithful to patients
who needed their care.

The second moral dilemma the nurses faced in working with
the "evil enemy" was the patients themselves. They were frightened. They hurt, in pain—in other words, human.

The prisoners of war seemed tired and fearful for their lives.
Many prisoners thought the nurses were trying to kill them. For
example, a Viet Cong patient who did not understand the treatment cried during a blood transfusion because he thought the
nurses were taking his life away. Enemy patients in full body
casts or lying on Stryker frame beds (a special bed used for
spinal cord injuries) would fall out of bed trying to escape from
what they thought were torture tactics rather than medical procedures.

The prisoner's fearful reactions made the nurses realize that
they too could be perceived as evil. Their technical skills and
their physical appearance—red and blond hair, freckles, and
height—made them appear strange and formidable to the Vietnamese. Military morality seemed absurd to the nurses who had
come to understand that both sides in the war were fearful of each
other. Fear was prohibiting the nurses and patients from accom-
plishing the basic task—to allow the patient to get well. Abol-
ishing this fear made the nurses' professional duties much easier.

Nurses watched the evil they thought so pervasive in enemy
soldiers disappear in the hospital wards. One nurse recalled a
prisoner on the ward who was shot through the neck. "Only his
eyes could move, not his head," she remembered. "He looked
dangerous and shifty. He bothered me because he followed me
with his eyes. One day he started to yell very loud. I couldn't
figure out what he was doing until I realized a child was climbing
over a crib rail and he was trying to warn me the kid was going to
fall and get hurt. After that I figured he was normal like everyone
else." It was difficult to hate someone who clearly felt the same
concern for children as the nurses did.

After two or three months in Vietnam, the majority of the nurses in the study (85 percent) looked on the enemy as patients in need of their care. As one army nurse said, "I came to realize, well, it's just their luck to be here. They [the enemy] are just patients and they deserve to be treated the same."

Five nurses in the study, however, were never able to work comfortably with either enemy or civilian Vietnamese. One of these nurses said, "It got to be very difficult working with the Vietnamese. We were fighting a culture. They'd rip out tubes and IVs. We were practicing voodoo as far as they were concerned. We had an interpreter trying to tell them we weren't going to hurt them. You could take that for just so long. I couldn't keep my temper." Four of the five requested and received transfers out of the wards with Vietnamese patients rather than show callousness and uncaring actions to the civilians. One nurse continued to work with them because her transfer request was denied. She decided to keep an emotional distance from the Vietnamese. She mechanically went about the daily routine. This nurse served her twelve-month tour but felt none of the satisfaction that comes from getting to know patients. To this day, she remains angry at the Vietnamese.

The nurses mentioned other medical personnel who shared this anger or who never changed their ideas about the evil enemy. Dealing with the prejudice of fellow nurses, doctors, and corpsmen was a new experience for many nurses who had to confront the idea that all health-care professionals were not universally humane with their care. One nurse, disgusted with the injustice she saw at her hospital, summed up the feelings of others who saw the enemy, and all Vietnamese, as human beings: "When you see a mother weeping for her dead child, that crosses all cultural and language barriers."

In the end, the nurses in the study resolved the moral dilemma. These women determined their professional nursing morals overruled any patriotic military morality.

A second moral quandary nurses faced in Vietnam was sending recuperated patients back to their fighting units. In order to maintain military troop strength, patients with minor injuries or illnesses were sent back to continue their combat duties. This action conflicted with another basic nursing moral: heal the patients and put them on a path to keep them healthy. "Watching the patients take off their pajamas, put on their fatigues, and climb into a boat that took them back to the war was very difficult," said a navy nurse. Everyone wondered when and if they would admit their young patients again. In a few instances, nurses recognized a name and saw a familiar face being readmitted for new wounds.

These situations set up a tension between the nurses' inner ideals and the outer reality of the war. The military procedure was logical but it set up feeling of confusion and guilt. The nurses wanted to say no to sending men back to combat but they realized they had no individual power to control or change the fate of their patients. They resolved this moral dilemma in a different manner from the tension posed by caring for enemy patients. Most nurses (88 percent of the sample) accepted the fact that, in war, the sense of free choice and individual beliefs was lost. Military orders silenced their inner voices. Nurses helped their patients recuperate and wished them well. They accepted the fact that some men would be wounded again and die. It was part of the cruel irony of war.

The nurses who could not accept this military dictum continued to feel guilty about their role in sending men back to combat. The powerlessness they felt turned to anger and this anger churned inside them. "I wanted to scream at the world," said one women. "This [war] was crazy and it had to stop." These women endured their wartime tours but returned home angry. Afterward, they used psychotherapy or supportive veterans, family, and friends to clear up their anxiety over this moral dilemma. They had acted against their beliefs. It was a difficult burden to bear.

4

The Rewards of Wartime Nursing in Vietnam

In Vietnam, nurses could easily become overwhelmed by work demands, fears, loneliness, and losses. But the same stress-filled world that produced so much strain also provided a balance. There was a rewarding side to the work and life in a war zone. The soldiers they helped heal, the feelings of being needed and appreciated, and, most importantly, the camaraderie that developed between nurses and other Americans helped individuals survive their wartime journeys.

The great majority of the patients, or course, recovered and their recoveries gave the nurses' tour a balance. Helping to save lives was the basic reason most nurses volunteered to go to Vietnam and, working with other medical personnel, they were very successful in achieving this objective. Ninety-eight percent of the wounded patients who entered military hospitals in Vietnam survived.[1] Nurses felt appreciated by the soldiers who seemed so grateful to have American women caring for them and their comrades. Nurses symbolized the protective, orderly way of life of the home the men yearned for. Watching the nurses work took some of the fear away from the patients who waited on a triage line for an operation or who rested in a bunk on a hospital ship that was rolling in the waves of the South China Sea. Soldiers even used a nickname—"round eyes"—to differentiate American and Vietnamese women.

Personal satisfaction was heightened by the knowledge that nurses were respected not only for their technical skills but for their clinical judgments as well.

During the time of the war, nurses back home were just beginning to establish themselves as an autonomous group.[2] Hospital and medical paternalism had a strong grip on the profession. Nurses took commands from physicians and were expected to do only as they were told. Vietnam was a different story. At war, there was little time for politics or sexist roles. If there was a decision to be made, it was taken for granted that the nurse would make it. Their skills were appreciated, their judgments about treatments and patients care were respected by their medical colleagues. "I never felt I was alone," said a nurse who recalled the decisions she had made as a twenty-three-year-old lieutenant in the receiving ward of a small surgical hospital south of Saigon. "I always knew I had support and a physician was nearby that I could count on."

One nurse said, "I'm not sure I've ever enjoyed nursing as much as I did that year. It was the most exciting, the most challenging, the most stressful, and the most important nursing practice I've ever done." This professional equality, however, did not continue once they returned home. Many nurses missed it and spent years searching for a clinical position where they could work as they had in Vietnam.

There were times when patients who were not expected to live overcame the odds and went home to recuperate among family and friends. Memories of unusual and dramatic recoveries remain vivid. Nurses learned that unanticipated events need not always be "bad." Charlie and John (pseudonyms) were patients who provided two memories.

Charlie was a blond nineteen-year-old soldier who had fractured both his femurs. The femur (or thigh bone) is the largest straight bone in the body. One of the complications that can occur after a large bone fracture is the release of fat emboli (or clots) from the broken bone into the blood stream. If these clots travel to the lungs and brain they result in a coma and death.[3] Recovery is uncertain. Charlie had a fat embolus. He was in a coma. The army nurse assigned to care for him was new to Vietnam. She was enthusiastic and anxious to prove her competence. "I wouldn't give up on him," she said. "Everyday I'd say 'Wake up Charlie, wake up.' Gradually, he came around and started talking to me. I felt like saying 'See, we can do it.' We shipped him home. I remember he had such clear blue eyes." Charlie taught this nurse a lesson she needed: that she was professionally competent and could handle the rigors of the work. He also showed her, and the other people who worked on her ward, that the human spirit was unpredictable and that her perseverance and patience with him were as important to his recovery as her skills with medical equipment.

John, an army corporal with the physical build of a football player, arrived at the twenty-fourth Evacuation Hospital in Long Binh unconscious. He had a severe head injury from an exploding land mine. John had the symptoms of a person who was about to die: his pupils would not constrict to light and his posture on the stretcher was decerebrate. (This term describes someone with stiff, unmoving extremities; it indicates massive brain damage.)[4] Physicians determined that John was an "expectant case" and ordered corpsmen to put him behind a curtain until he died. They moved him to the back of the receiving ward and began the sad routine. "I was taking his pulse and the corpsman was cleaning the mud off him," recalled the nurse on duty that day. "The corpsman was quietly talking to the patient. He said, 'What do you want for breakfast, John?' Well, from under this huge bandage a voice says, 'A chocolate milk shake.' The corpsmen turn white. I get a surgeon. They remove a hematoma [blood clot] from John's brain. He had hemiplegia [partial paralysis] but at least he goes home alive." The nurse and corpsmen often spoke about John. He became a symbol of triumph among the other lost young men.

Other nurses found rewards in less dramatic ways. The women enjoyed simply talking to their patients. Usually, at night, when the frantic pace slowed down, they would listen to their patients' stories about home and their plans for home. Patients often talked about girl friends and wives, their relationships, their problems. Because they were American women the nurses were viewed as available experts on matters of the heart.

A nurse who worked the night shift at the sixty-seventh Evacuation Hospital remembered a soldier whose leg was amputated. He asked the nurse for help in writing a letter home to his wife to tell her about his disfigurement. How could he go home without a leg? What did she think his wife would feel or say? Over several nights, until his transfer to another hospital, the two of them talked. A few months later, the nurse, who still worked the night shift in Vietnam, received a thank-you from the soldier. It was a picture of him, with his wife—skiing, back in his home state of Colorado.

Navy nurses on the hospital ships remembered their young marine patients who never forgot military jargon and etiquette no matter how inappropriate it was to the situation. For example, one patient woke from surgery, saw a set of lieutenant's bars on a nurse's collar, and came to attention on his stretcher. Another patient would hold up a sign for arriving wounded patients that read: "Pain builds character," no doubt a reminder of the famous Marine Corps image of emotional and physical strength. The men would laugh as they were wheeled into a treatment room for wound cleaning and suturing.

Friends made the work go smoothly. Nurses could count on a friend to do a job correctly. Friends also helped ease the sense of isolation and loneliness that often closed in during quiet hours after work. What was unexpected about the friendships formed in Vietnam was the intense nature of these relationships. More than half of the nurses (55 percent) reported that their social relationships in Vietnam were among the most intimate of their lives. As one nurse said, "I don't think I have ever been as close to people as I was in Vietnam. I became friends with people I probably wouldn't have met at home. I couldn't have made it through that year without them."

Isolated from contact with the rest of their world, nurses turned to their wartime friends to meet the needs normally satisfied by family and friends back home. Nurses needed to feel recognition, approval, and in general an appreciation for themselves as human beings. There were fewer people to meet their

needs, so those who were available became even more important. Friends formed groups and groups became "families."
These families helped nurses feel protected and needed in the
environment of war. A sentimental, intense kind of love developed between friends.[5] This intensity remained strong and, for
many, has never been duplicated.

There was more opportunity to become close to people because the usual barriers to friendship that existed back in the
United States did not exist in Vietnam. Everyone lived in the
same quarters. There was no hierarchy between higher and lower
ranking officers. Colonels and captains lived in the same type of
room or ship's cabin as lieutenants. Military law confined everyone to small areas. No one was allowed to leave any military
compound without permission and often an armed guard. Such
confinement meant there were always people available in the
ward room, officers' quarter, or "hooches" to talk or relax with
after work.

Everyone had the same sense of mission—to save lives. This
common goal made the family of friends more significant than any
other relationship. Morale was often tied in with the group friendships. A friendly, cohesive group kept a sad, lonely person strong
while a dispirited group could undermine a stable person.

In the army and air force everyone dressed in the same
combat fatigue uniform. Money meant nothing. Military scrip
replaced dollars and the difference in pay from rank to rank was
slight. There was very little available that their salaries could
buy; thus, it was a woman's emotional capital that determined
who her friends were.

To the nurses, the most supportive people in their world were
fellow nurses. There was an emotional and intellectual affinity
between those women who worked and lived together. A room-
mate or a staff nurse from the same hospital unit made a good
confidante. Who better to understand the depths of a nurse's
feelings than someone who faced the same thoughts in the same
world? Just as they comforted their patients, nurses helped each
other.

Living quarters resembled college dormitories when a group
of off-duty nurses got together to share a food package from
home. An unwritten rule of friendship was: whatever belonged to

one belonged to all. The women listened to each other as they cooked pizza in frying pans or made packaged macaroni and cheese. They closed themselves off from the war and drew from each other.

A few friendships outlasted the war. Fifteen years later, for example, two navy nurses had who served side by side in Vietnam on a hospital ship arrived together for the study interview. Their friendship has lasted through graduate school, marriages, cross country moves, children, and many different jobs. Why these two women remained friends is uncertain. They simply made the effort to stay in touch. Clearly fond of each other, the two have a friendship that is one of the few lasting rewards from the war.

There were others among the American forces the nurses counted as friends. Three of the nurses included military chaplains in their Vietnam families. Most of the women, however, mentioned physicians, corpsmen, technicians or medics, and the helicopter pilots who brought wounded patients in from the field as comprising their main group of friends. Physicians and pilots held the same military rank as the nurses. It was acceptable, by military code, and convenient to talk and socialize with these men. Helicopter pilots were generally single and the same age as the nurses.

Some friendships developed into romances, others remained platonic. A few marriages and lifelong friendships evolved from these wartime relationships. One physician-nurse team became particularly faithful friends. They met in 1965 as part of a group of medical military officers assigned to help Vietnamese nurses upgrade surgical operating room techniques in a small provincial hospital near the Gulf of Thailand. He was the surgeon. She was the operating room nurse. They worked side-by-side for a year and then came home to different careers and families. She stayed single and had a successful military career. He pursued his surgical work, but their friendship remained strong. Every Sunday morning for the last twenty years, this nurse has received a telephone call from him. He calls her to say hello to see how she is doing.

The nurses spoke most fondly of the enlisted men who worked with them. Different services gave different titles to these men: in the air force they were called "technicians," in the navy "corpsmen," and in the army "medics." They worked closely with the nurses on the evacuation planes, in hospital units, and on ships. At work, the nurses could not survive without them. Experienced corpsmen helped nurses new to their profession and the war learn essential skills. During busy times, corpsmen assumed more clinical responsibility and assisted the nurses in getting wounded patients treated quickly.

During quiet times, corpsmen turned to the nurses for advice. Although they were officers, nurses were considered approachable because they were so near in age to the enlisted men. Showing interest and concern for their corpsmen was not an unselfish deed for the nurses. They received attention and satisfaction in return. Nurses could offer these enlisted men little more than a compassionate ear. Senior nurses, who were in position to recommend promotions, were not able to reward the enlisted men they admired so much. One nurse who supervised the entire nursing staff on a hospital ship said, "The corpsmen were outstanding but we couldn't get them promoted. We could only promote people within the nurse corps, which was frustrating. The corpsmen who worked on the line [with the troops] got easier promotions. The only way we could recognize them was giving the time off and giving them small awards when they left [to go home]."

Five nurses in the study preferred the off-duty company of enlisted men. They felt more comfortable with men nearer in age who shared their interest in music, food, and politics. Physicians were usually older than the nurses and usually married. Becoming friendly off-duty with corpsmen could be a source of stress. It was against military code for officers to fraternize with enlisted personnel, and if they were discovered everyone would be punished.[6] "I had to watch my step," said a nurse who later married a corpsman, "because I would have gotten into trouble." Despite the frequent stories nurses told about dating enlisted men, no one in the study was disciplined for these actions.

According to the nurses, the military command made it difficult to maintain friendships. All military personnel had individual arrival and departure dates exactly 365 days apart. Most people came and left Vietnam alone. It was not unusual for a nurse to become friendly with people only to watch them "rotate" out of the unit or ship and return home. Several nurses said, "You got tired of saying good-bye." Once the friendship breaks up, who was there to rely on? The benefit of the long-term camaraderie that was experienced in previous wars, when whole units traveled to and from a war zone together, was missing in the Vietnam War.[7]

In spite of the constant changes in personnel, wartime friendships remained stronger—whether it was in building barbecue patios next to living quarters, having water fights during the monsoon season, putting together variety shows on the ship's deck, or talking in a quiet place.

One nurse summed up the feelings of all the other nurses when she said, "My true brothers and sisters were the people I was with in Vietnam."

5
Personal Experiences in Vietnam

Even though they did not fight battles, the nurses saw the need to develop survival skills. Survival was more than living through enemy attacks. It was a need to preserve emotional and personal integrity in a world where people were torn loose from community and home moorings.

Friends helped one another, but each nurse came to realize she had to cope with wartime stresses alone. Friends became involved in their own concerns. Friends went home. Friends became casualties.

Sometimes, men they socialized with, or, in two instances, husbands and men they planned to marry, were killed. Most of the casualties the nurses knew were helicopter pilots who shared their work and off-duty time. Pilots had common ground with nurses. Both groups were young and single and worked with the wounded.

Seven nurses recalled times when a pilot was declared missing. It would be early evening at the officers' club. People arrived after work for the daily happy hour of drinks, talk, and music.

Nurses, physicians, pilots, and other officers mingled around the bar and nearby tables. A familiar face would not appear and word quickly spread that John and Bob or Bill or Charlie had been shot down. The loud bar banter became quieter. A normal day in the war became grim and empty of meaning.

Prior to going to Vietnam, few people had thought about the possibility of dying. To dwell on such thoughts would make it difficult, most likely impossible, to climb on aircraft flying to Saigon or Da Nang. Friends spent time talking about the heat and where they hoped to be stationed. Anyone with thoughts and fears about injury or death kept quite. But this prewar naiveté seemed frivolous once the casualty count with familiar names started to rise.

The futility of this stateside innocence became evident to one army nurse shortly after she arrived in Vietnam. She spoke about getting a telegram one day while she worked in the twelfth Evacuation Hospital's receiving ward in Cu Chi.

I was stationed at Fort Bragg before Vietnam. I was close to a guy from the eighty-second Airborne Division. We weren't close like boy friend and girl friend. He was like a younger brother, probably the same age as my brother back home. He took out a fifty-thousand-dollar life insurance policy on himself before he left and I get this check for fifty-thousand dollars when I'm in 'Nam because he dies over there and I was his beneficiary. I had to get his parents' address. I didn't want this money. It was a big laugh when we were in North Carolina but it wasn't a laugh now that this nineteen-year-old guy is dead. I didn't care what they did with the money but I wasn't taking any of it.

She found his parents and forwarded the check to them.

Not all stories about missing pilots ended with sadness. A former army nurse who now lives in suburban New Jersey with her husband and children told a remarkable tale about a man she knew in Vietnam while she was stationed at the sixty-seventh Evacuation Hospital in Qui Nhon during 1967 and 1968. "We used to party with the helicopter pilots," she said while we sat in her kitchen on a hot June day.

They ate in our mess hall. One guy I was friendly with was very excited about his upcoming baby [a boy was born back home]. Then I didn't see him for about two weeks. I asked one of the other pilots what happened to him. They said his helicopter was shot down and they think he's a prisoner. I never heard any more. In 1971, I was married and living in Denver and watching the release of the prisoners of war. Damned if he wasn't one of them! I went to see him and he told me he relived those days at the sixty-seventh Evac so many times in prison.

Two nurses lost men they loved. One women's husband was killed in Vietnam before she reached her overseas assignment. When she arrived at her assignment in Cu Chi, she asked the chief nurse not to tell anyone about his death. "I didn't want anyone's pity or anyone to say 'Oh, I'm sorry.'" She occupied herself with work and friends. Perhaps, she thought, she could help save another woman's husband.

Six months into her tour, she transferred to a larger evacuation hospital at Long Binh. She fell in love again. He was a helicopter pilot. Her life seemed to be better. She could see a future for herself. Two months before she was due to come home, a young terrorist pulled a grenade and killed himself and the pilot.

She cried as she spoke of both men: "After he [the pilot] died, I said, 'The hell with relationships. This is for the birds.' You reach out to someone and then they are lost." Her voice was melancholy, not bitter. She came home alone, and remained single. Today she runs her own successful health care business but she says she still thinks of her losses.

While the nurses in the study freely spoke about everything that happened to them in Vietnam, a personal loss was different from a professional loss because the nurse could not easily hide behind a stiff exterior. The grief was real.

Another nurse, whose fiancé died in Vietnam, said his death shaped her life. I heard her story from other women in June 1984 during the week I interviewed a number of nurses who had served together on the USS *Repose*. Each brought it up. The man was a line officer involved in the daily routine of keeping the hospital ship fit for sea.

The naval officer and I were in the middle of the interview when she shifted in her chair and said, "I guess you've heard about Jack [a pseudonym]."

We were the good in the midst of all this carnage and blood and pain. We planned to be married. My tour ended first so I went home and he was transferred from the ship to Vietnam. He was killed on the tenth day of our separation. I got the telegram and it was devastating. There is a whole time period [after the telegram] that I don't remember. I know I went to work but I couldn't tell you what I did. I went right back to work [after Vietnam] because I was saving time to be with him.

My parents were so excited. They never thought I'd marry and be domestic. They never got to meet him.

I was a lieutenant in my late twenties and I had a great number of experiences. Here I met this man who, compared to the men before him and after him, well, he was the epitome.

After he died, it became extremely important for me to find out what happened to him. I had this sense that if I just could have been there I could have done something. Of course this wasn't realistic but I still felt this way. I did find the corpsman who was with him when he died. I learned Jack was at a supply depot that got hit. He was alert and conscious after he'd been hit with a mortar round. Jack tried to help his buddy. The [evacuation] chopper he was put on crashed! He was finally taken to a battalion aid station but he died en route. I figured out that what happened was that he was caught in the confusion and the up-heaval in the triage system during Tet [the major military offensive of 1968]. There was a seven-hour delay from the time he was hit until he got to battalion aid. I kept thinking, if he'd gotten to the ship [the USS *Repose*] . . . I didn't accept his death for a long time. I thought the phone was going to ring because I'd heard stories about mix-ups.

My friends from the ship helped me get through this period. They stuck with me and I'm not the kind of person who reaches out much. In order to keep on going physically, you get over the pain but you never completely forget it. I never could have lived with that kind of pain.

It's obvious I've never married. It's hard to compete with a ghost.

She did not cry, nor did she seem self-pitying. She said she misses Jack and the life they might have shared. She has, as psychologists who study bereavement say, "worked through" his death.[1] It is a difficult process that can take years, and sometimes psychological help, to accomplish.

Unlike this navy nurse, an air force nurse who lost two friends in Vietnam is still trying to make sense of their deaths. The unusual aspect of her story is that her friends were women.

Air force nurses with flying assignments in South Vietnam got to know the country. It was not unusual for them to land at ten different places in one day as they ferried patients from battlefield to hospital. There were opportunities to meet people. She was happy to talk with the two women because she was the only female in her squadron and she missed the companionship of women. One of the women she met was a nurse from California, the other a lab technician from Australia. "Both women were in Vietnam with Project Concern, a voluntary civilian organization that provided health care and other services to the South Vietnamese," the air force nurse said. The three women got together whenever they could. She brought them underwear from the PX. They gave her locally grown strawberries. They became close friends.

One night, the air force nurse got a call from her commander. "He told me the VC had overrun the [Project Concern] hospital and killed everyone who was there. Including my two friends. I was devastated. They were my only female friends. I couldn't mourn and be sad because I had to get up and go to work the next day. Crying wouldn't do me any good." This air force nurse eventually went into counseling, a treatment recommended by psychologists who work with veterans.[2] I saw her again two years after the research interview. She told me, "I'm so much better now."

The deaths of the two civilian women exposed the arbitrariness of wartime violence. Men died in combat and battle but no one expected women to die. It seemed the height of unreason and madness.

There are no exact figures for American civilian deaths in the Vietnam War. Various organizations like the Red Cross compile numbers but a comprehensive picture is not available. In contrast, the military has precise records on nurses who died. Journalists chronicled their deaths.[3] Official records indicate that eight female and two male nurses died as a result of illness or injury sustained in Vietnam.[4]:

- One nurse, 1st Lt. Sharon Lane, died on June 8, 1969, at the three-hundred-and-twelfth Evacuation Hospital in Chu Lai as the result of fatal shrapnel wounds from enemy fire. She is the only female military nurse killed by hostile fire in the Vietnam War.
- Two army nurses, 2nd Lt. Carol Ann Drazba and 2d Lt. Elizabeth Ann Jones, were killed on February 18, 1966, near Saigon in a helicopter crash. Lieutenant Jones's fi-

ancé, Lt. Col. Charles M. Honour, piloted the helicopter. He died with her.

· On November 30, 1967, near Qui Nhon, two female army nurses, Capt. Eleanor Alexander and 1st Lt. Hedwig Orlowski, died in a plane crash that also killed two male nurses, 1st Lt. Jerome Olmstead and 1st Lt. Kenneth Shoemaker, Jr.

· 2d Lt. Pamela Donovan died of pneumonia on July 8, 1968, at the eighty-fifth Evacuation Hospital in Qui Nhon, where she was stationed.

· Lt. Col. Annie Ruth Graham, who served with the Army Nurse Corps during World War II and in the Korean War, suffered a stroke at the ninety-first Evacuation Hospital when it was located in Tuy Hoa. She was flown for treatment to Japan where she died on August 14, 1968.

· One air force nurse, Capt. Mary Klinker, was killed in Operation Babylift—an effort to bring orphans to the United States at the end of the war. The plane crash that killed her, ten other crew members, and 144 passengers on April 9, 1975 also injured four other air force nurses.

Many nurses developed a professional veneer in order to face each day. The practice has its origins in the teachings of Florence Nightingale, who established the Nightingale School for the training nurses in 1860. She wrote that the young women in her program must refrain from displaying any emotions in their work. Such strictness was necessary to overcome the prevailing views that equated nursing with scouring maids and prostitutes. Nightingale felt that nurses must not allow themselves to be women. They must be professional people. In an early essay advocating formal training for nurses, Nightingale wrote, "You do not want the effect of your good things to be 'How wonderful for a women!' . . . you want to do the thing that is good whether it is suitable for a woman or not."[5] Helpless Victorian women who wrung their hands at the slightest pressure and who needed men to make even the most minute decisions had no place in Nightingale's world.[6]

Repression of emotion came to haunt some nurses after they returned stateside because it prevented them from venting pent-up feelings, but in Vietnam the stiff exterior had been an effective way to cope with all the suffering. By insulating themselves—building a shield—nurses avoided feeling sad or angry or helpless. They were able to do the jobs that had to be done. An army nurse who worked in the receiving ward of the twelfth Evacuation hospital near the Cambodian border remembered "not getting overly emotional with patients, just in case they died. You did not want to get too attached to them. We had to do that in order to keep going."

It amazed some nurses that they never cried in Vietnam. These women cry today over the same scenes and people. For them, the need to be tough ended with the war. By coming home they could begin to let themselves feel.

Nurses did not arrive in Vietnam with plans to hide their emotions. Gradually, they started to feel a change in their own behavior. "Patients," as one nurse said, "were no longer people. They were wounds to me. They were heads and backs. I never thought I'd say that, but it happened. The more patients we lost, the less I wanted to know. If someone died, well, they'd bring in five more patients."

Some nurses learned to selectively avoid patients, especially those men who were going to die. Concentrating on the living made it easier to work each day. Some nurses stopped reading the *Stars and Stripes* (the daily military paper that extensively covered the war) because the names in the "Killed in Action" column often were former patients or friends. With the day equally divided into twelve hours shifts, there was no time to dwell on sadness.

To the uninitiated, these women may have seemed hard, but those who came to know them saw a different picture. A navy nurse who worked in the operating rooms of the USS *Repose* remembered a head nurse who had the reputation of running the orthopedic ward of the ship with an iron hand.

It looked like she had no compassion for the guys [patients]. Actually, she was all heart but she just didn't show it. I learned about her other side through our washing machines! We had two machines on board that we used to clean clothes. Every time I would go down to use them there would be marine fatigues in the machine. I couldn't figure out what was going on. Well, this women told me she bought soap and after shave lotion and when the marine pilots would drop off patients she would ask them if they wanted a shower and shave before going back to the field [jungle]. She'd wash their uniforms while they showered. And this was the woman who was tough as nails.

Soon, I started doing the same thing. I'd say to the marines who brought in the casualties, 'Hey kid, do you want to take a shower?' We started keeping towels for them. The commanding officer of the ship was always complaining about our use of water. He never knew.

Some nurses were not as successful as others in developing a tough exterior. These women were usually young and new to the war. At night, after work, they sat on the helipad outside a hospital or stood on the ship's deck at sunset and cried. Some cried themselves to sleep thinking of the patients in their wards and of those who died. Each death became a personal failure. Feelings of inadequacy mounted and became overpowering. They tried to make sense out of the senseless. Unless a concerned friend stepped in to help her overcome her helplessness, a nurse could easily become an emotional victim of the war. The longer she was in the war, the more she tried to hide from her feelings by becoming reclusive and not socializing. Or she hid from herself with drinking, and drugs.

When work was over for the day, nurses learned to rest. Relaxation took many forms in Vietnam. The nurses and the people they worked with relaxed with the same energy they put into work. Everything in wartime had a compulsiveness that was seldom found in peacetime. Work was intense. Relaxation was intense. People filled officers' clubs and planned parties for the slightest excuse. Many military groups had monthly "Hail and Farewell" parties for newcomers and veterans going home. The parties were a respite, a chance to leave the anguish. Everyone drank, danced, and sang songs. In 1969, many women remembered singing a popular song by a group called The Animals: "We Gotta Get Out Of This Place." The chorus contained the line: "If it's this last thing we ever do." The singing and laughter temporarily masked the truthful message of the song.

Nurses who did not like parties often enjoyed watching movies in the mess hall or on the flight deck. When mail deliveries slowed, people watched the same movie night after night. At the ninety-fifth Evacuation Hospital in Da Nang, "The Good, the Bad and the Ugly," a Clint Eastwood Western, had twenty-two consecutive showings. Others preferred quieter activities. They decorated their living quarters to resemble home. These nurses made curtains, bedspreads, and afghans. Some nurses preferred academic work and took correspondence courses from home. One woman became an expert on tropical diseases. Two nurses went to Catholic Mass every day.

Sending letters and cassette tapes home was another off-duty exercise. Thinking about their families reminded people the war would end. There was a world waiting for them. Just as nurses felt a responsibility to protect and to comfort their patients, they felt a responsibility to home. Every nurse in the study mentioned writing only positive messages home. There was no need to worry parents and friends. Writing about only the excitement and the good times was an escape. Good news, they though, would relieve parents of any of the anxiety or guilt they felt about having their daughters in the war. Most parents saved the letters or tapes but more than half of the nurses have never looked or listened to them. The women who have read their letters noticed how young they were when they wrote them. The prose is filled with exclamation points and words like "hi" with the dot of the "i" a smiling face. Others have not looked at their messages because they worry that reading them may bring back unwanted memories.

No matter what the activity, nurses tried to spend little time alone. The emotional shield nurses constructed to cope with the stress would disintegrate with too much introspection. War gave loneliness a special meaning. An army nurse who worked in the intensive care unit at the seventy-first Evacuation Hospital near the mountains of Pleiku remembered "a different kind of lonely feeling. Maybe hollow. I think back to some of the relationships and things I did and it was this incredible attempt to fill an ever deepening empty space inside. Everything I believed—my idealism, my romanticism, my faith—was destroyed." For her and others, the war altered values as well as people.

But despite any inner changes, the nurses still had to report for duty. It seemed wise to avoid unsettling thoughts. The nurses innately sensed that Vietnam was not the place to ponder their changed view of the world. Their energies were needed on the work units. They could not leave the war when they tired of it. The question "What's happened to me?" needed to be pushed aside and into the future. Keeping busy on and off duty was the best way to postpone self-analysis. "I came back to my room at seven o'clock," said another woman. "I hopped in the shower, got dressed and went somewhere just to be with people. You didn't spend much time alone and I'm wondering if it was because you didn't want to."

The culture of war dictated new rules and new behaviors. One widely held rule was to relax quickly at the end of the workday. Drinking was the most common way to unwind. Seventy-five percent of the nurses in the study mentioned drinking as the preferred way to slow down after work. Those women who never drank at home because of religious beliefs or parental rules found themselves in a bar drinking a beer or martini after work. Liquor was cheap and available everywhere, even on the ships, where it was supposedly forbidden. The cost of a case of beer was the same as the cost of a case of Coca Cola. Most people would stop by the officers' club for a few drinks before heading to the mess hall or quarters for dinner with friends. During the research interviews, some nurses smiled when they recalled how much they drank and others voiced surprise at it, but none of the nurses apologized for drinking. It was acceptable wartime behavior.

So too was the use of drugs, especially marijuana, accepted as another way to relax. Vietnam was the first war in which military personnel admitted to illegal drug use.[7] Drugs such as marijuana, hashish, opium, and heroin were widely available. People used drugs for the same reason they used alcohol, to relax and to escape from the war. Some young nurses were familiar with the drug culture flourishing back home. For them, marijuana was as acceptable a way to unwind as liquor was to older nurses. Four nurses said they regularly smoked marijuana with their friends. "Initially, I drank a lot but I couldn't deal with the hangovers," said a woman, "That's when I started to use marijuana. We'd sit around, listen to music, and get high." If caught using drugs, these women would be sent home for military discipline and also face the possible loss of their nursing license. Yet they did not worry about the chance they were taking. The risk of death and the unpleasantness of the war made them immune to legal codes. "What are they going to do with me? Send me to Vietnam?" they asked.

Alcohol and drugs may have provided a needed escape during the war but using them at home to hide from memories only postponed inevitable confrontations with the past. Two women continued to smoke marijuana and risk legal trouble in the 1970s. As they matured and married and had children, drugs became less suited to their lifestyles. One turned to group counseling with other veterans in order to deal with her memories. The other still uses drugs but claims she no longer thinks about the war.

Seven nurses said they drank from the time they got off duty in Vietnam until light out. They drank to numb their minds from thoughts of work. Two nurses became alcoholics. For these women, alcohol and Vietnam became one. That is, they could not drink without thinking of the war and the war made them drink. Caught in a destructive spiral, they had to sort out their feelings before they could successfully stop drinking. Many years after the war, both joined Alcoholics Anonymous. Members in this organization provided the support the women needed to stop their abuse. One of the nurses had started drinking heavily at the age of twenty-three in Vietnam and became sober when she was thirty-five years old. Looking back, she said recovering from alcoholism was probably as difficult as some of her patients' rehabilitation from physical war wounds.

6

The Status of Female Military Nurses in Vietnam

There is a maldistribution of the sexes in war. Combat and war are masculine experiences. No one is sure of the total number of nurses who served in Vietnam, but estimates indicate they were a small minority in the overall American effort.[1] Their needs seemed inconsequential. Official emphasis was on combat, tactics, and men.

Military leaders knew women were serving in Vietnam.[2] But they did little to provide them with the necessities. For example, the military PX stores located on the bases where the nurses lived carried soap and shampoo but not tampons. These same stores carried nylon stockings, but, as one nurse said, "we didn't have a great need for nylons with our fatigues. They were probably there for the soldiers to buy for their local girl friends." Military women were almost invisible, while women who filled traditional roles in war—the barmaid, the prostitute—were not.

The nurses learned in this overwhelmingly male environment and came to view the lack of planning for women with a mixture of disbelief and humor. Most of the oversights concerning women were merely embarrassing or uncomfortable.

An army lieutenant learned about being a minority when she contracted food poisoning and found herself in a medical ward filled with male patients. It was a communal existence. "I remember," she said, "even sharing the bathroom! I found myself sitting [in the bathroom] next to a man. We'd all shuffle in with our IVs, hang them on the toilet door, weakly smile at each other, and later shuffle out." How did she feel about this privation? At first she was so sick she did not care who saw her, but later, when her sense of propriety returned, she wondered why there was only one women's bathroom in the whole hospital. Perhaps military leaders never thought women would get sick or need bathrooms at work.

Then there was a group of nurses who realized the standard issue metal helmets did not fit a woman's head covered in hair curlers! "It became a big joke with us [the nurses]," said a former lieutenant. "When the alert siren went off, we had to decide if we were really going to get hit so you could rip out your curlers." The longer they spent in Vietnam, the more accurate their assessments of the alert situations. No one wanted to waste valuable sleeping time on unnecessary grooming. The nurses had never imagined they would blend the art of hairstyles with helmets and sirens.

But there were occasions when the oversight and narrow thinking of military planners proved potentially dangerous. Throughout Vietnam, troops had prepared for enemy attacks. Soldiers built bunkers, uncoiled concertina wire around base perimeters, and set up defense guns. Every soldier became familiar with the procedure to be followed when a "red alert" (warning of enemy attack) occurred. Veterans learned to be particularly watchful at night, the enemy's favorite time to lob mortars or send rockets crashing into the bases. Nurses received instructions on the procedures to be followed when the alarm sounded. Initially, all military personnel followed the same directives. But the "alert" orders for some women soon changed.

It was decided because there were only thirty of us [nurses] in this big base of men, it was probably dangerous to let us run out in our pajamas and nightgowns into the bunkers. Not dangerous in the sense that the enemy was going to get us but that the American men would see us. So the enlisted men sandbagged our Quonset huts [living quarters] to chest height. When we had an alert we were told to roll out of our bunks, put on flak [protective] jackets and helmets, and go under the bunk with our heads against the sandbags.

On paper, the alert procedure made sense, but the planners had neglected to consider female shape. "They didn't realize with the beds so low to the ground, if you had any bust at all you couldn't put your flak jacket on and get under the bed. You wouldn't fit! So what you did was crawl under the bunk and throw the jacket over yourself." None of the nurses in this group were injured.

At another military base, instead of trained military guards, medical corpsmen secured the nurses' compound. The corpsmen were not known for their proficiency with weapons. Fortunately, they were never called on to use them.

These stories illustrated three aspects about women in Vietnam. First, maintaining a sense of humor was important. Second, as a group nurses did not challenge foolish orders; they modified or worked around them. Third, military strategists seemed more interested in protecting women from their male comrades than from the enemy.

Yet these same authorities valued the nurses' professional skills. For this reason, chief nurses informed their staffs that, contrary to their impressions, nurses' lives were more important than soldiers' and that if a decision needed to be made during an attack, between saving an patient and saving a nurse, one should save the latter. "It seemed," said a nurse who remembered this order, "that everyone else was expendable but us." This policy also forbade nurses from riding in helicopters or driving jeeps and trucks.

The majority of the women chose not to think about this policy. It unsettled them to think that anyone was considered expendable, an idea that ran counter to their professional beliefs.

As officers, the nurses outranked many of the American men overseas. Most enlisted personnel, however, held a traditional view of women: they needed to be protected. In return, they expected the nurses to become surrogate mothers, sisters, wives, and girl friends. Thus an unwritten rule in Vietnam was: Men protected women; women, in turn, comforted the men.

Generally, the nurses were treated very well. They slept on beds or bunks, ate hot meals, and took (cold) showers. Supply sergeants often "found" valuable items like rain jackets and blankets for the women while the men stayed wet and cold.

Being protected by men and living in such a male world was both welcome and suffocating. Women had to be "on duty" twenty-four hours a day. Armed escorts accompanied the nurses every time they went off base. One nurse stopped going to orphanages when she realized a soldier might get wounded or killed defending her need to go off base. If there was a pool or beach near the hospital, nurses would gather three or four friends because they felt uneasy sitting alone in a bathing suit surrounded by two hundred men. The nurses who lived in Phu Bai, on the northern seacoast of South Vietnam, avoided the main base swimming pool, preferring a pool at the Special Forces camp down the road where there were never more than eight or ten men present. On the hospital ships, certain sun decks were reserved for the nurses. A woman always wore a shirt or some other cover-up while walking up to the deck to relax. Army nurses could not sit outside their quarters without men stopping their trucks to take pictures. When a woman walked into a PX store, the usual buzz of conversation stopped. Some men would stare, while other approached to talk. Initially, nurses enjoyed this attention, but it soon became restrictive because it invaded the women's privacy and their ability to unwind. There was no escape.

Sometimes, patients turned to nurses for the advice they normally sought from a sister or mother. The nurses' ability to comfort injured men was rewarding. One night in the summer of 1968, for example, an army nurse was checking her patients. Most of them had gone off to sleep. A young soldier, who had just lost an eye, got up to go to the bathroom. She thought he looked upset and asked him if he wanted to play a game of chess. As they sat around the game board, she asked him if something was bothering him. He said, "Yeah, from a woman's viewpoint, what do you think would be better, an artificial eye or a patch?"

Looking at him, she understood how important his appearance would be when he returned home and began dating. She knew nurses ignored the sight of bandages but young civilian women would quickly notice his injury. This nineteen-year-old veteran wanted to be handsome again. The nurse thought a moment and told him, "Gee, I always thought eye patches were daring but why don't you get both?" He looked at her and said, "Yeah, that's what I'm going to do." He finished playing the game and went back to sleep.

Even in androgynous fatigue uniforms, the nurses knew that patients never mistook them for men. Their physical size or their movements identified them to the men waiting to be moved from the battlefields to hospitals. Infantrymen lifted their wounded comrades into air force evacuation planes. As soon as the nurses came over to check their injuries, the wounded would ask them to hold their hands for a minute. Nurses frequently heard them say, "It just feels so good to touch someone." Touching an American woman made them feel secure and alive when so much else seemed uncertain.

But it was impossible to appear neat in 120 degree heat. Still, neither her dress nor the effect of the tropical heat on her appearance diminished a woman's presence to combat troops. One nurse, who sat in a research interview looking very professional in her tailored military uniform embellished with gold braid and three rows of medals, remembered a time in the war when she was not so polished:

I was in a mess tent eating dinner with a few other nurses and a group of marines. Everyone just wanted to hear us say, "Hello, how are you?" and "Things are fine with me, what about you?" We were sitting there eating. It was so hot and here we are in full uniform with girdles and stockings! I was sweating like a pig and every time I moved I heard click, click, click. I couldn't figure out what was happening. Finally I realized it was the guys taking our pictures. I asked them why they were bothering because we looked so disheveled! They said, "We haven't seen a 'round eye' in six months." A wilted uniform seemed unimportant.

It was difficult not to be flattered, and the nurses took their role as a symbol of home very seriously. They made an effort to stay as orderly and well-groomed as possible. They reported to work with their hair brushed and make-up in place. They smiled and spoke kindly to their patients and other men they visited. By today's standards, these measures might seem superficial and demeaning, so that the nurses appeared to be sex objects rather than professionals. In Vietnam, however, the nurses did not feel that way. Instead, they saw themselves as being able to provide temporary refuge from the brutal war. They extended the professional's desire and responsibility "to care" beyond their patients to all men at war who felt the need for comfort.

"There were so few American girls, we felt somewhat obliged to appear at parties," said a nurse who regularly attended social functions in Saigon. For some women, especially younger nurses who had rarely dated before the war, the social demands boosted their egos. Men always wanted to talk, to dance, or to buy them drinks. Physical looks were unimportant, the women could pick and choose with whom they spent their time. Being surrounded by men reminded one nurse of a popular series of movies from the early 1960s where innocent teen-age girls were chased by boys. "I felt like Annette Funicello in *Beach Party Bingo*."

Three women who served in Vietnam at different times saw an exploitative side to being invited to parties and other social functions. In one instance, a woman worked on a base where the commander of an army division periodically invited nurses to his air conditioned trailer for dinner. They ate off real plates instead of mess hall metal. Enlisted men served the meal. The nurses were told to dress in "real" dresses instead of their uniforms. This nurse went once to these functions and refused to go again. "I knew they were trying to be nice and give us a decent meal, but nonetheless I felt like a commodity. It was so chauvinistic. I said I'd be happy to go again if they invited the male nurses and some of the doctors." Providing diversion for high-ranking officers did not fit into her idea of supporting American men. Sitting in air conditioning and drinking fine wine was much different from sweating in a Marine Corps mess hall.

Quiet, shy women had a difficult time around the men. Going for a drink after work invariably involved talking, whether the woman wanted to or not. A twenty-one-year-old nurse learned this lesson one day when she ordered a beer and went to sit alone to read her mail and write an letter. "A warrant officer came up to me," she said, "and chewed me out for not being a socialite. He told me I owed it to these boys. I felt so guilty."

None of the nurses interviewed reported overt instances of sexual harassment. Two women mentioned taking specific measures to avoid problems. One nurse wore her fatigues as a defense. She felt if she wore a dress or other feminine clothes men would take advantage of her. Another nurse quickly got involved with a male officer because she sensed this would insulate her from any sexual pressures a single, unattached nurse might feel. Most of the women, however, shared the feelings of an army nurse who said, "Most of the guys were very sweet. There was very little in the way of what you would call sexual harassment. A few times, guys put 'the make' on you but when I let them know I was not interested, they left me alone."

In 1984, Paul and O'Neill conducted a survey of 137 nurses who served in Vietnam. The results of their study showed different responses to questions of sexual harassment. They wrote that 63 percent of the nurses in their sample reported some form of sexual harassment while in Vietnam. These incidents ranged from pranks (using women's underwear as an antenna flag) to serious (threats of military discipline if a woman would not sleep with a high-ranking officer).[2] The difference in the nurses' responses may be due to the way in which this subject was approached. Paul and O'Neill prominently and explicitly asked questions about sexual harassment in their questionnaire. In the current study, the question was more implicit. Discussion about intimidation was likely to occur when the nurses responded to the question: "American women were certainly a minority in Vietnam. Did this fact have any effect on the way you could relax or cope with all the stress around you?"

Sexual harassment was not confined to the military in wartime. Women in uniform continue to experience it. A 1987 report submitted to the Defense Department found that sexual mistreatment "is alive and well today."[3] In a world where men are trained to use intimidation to fight and to maintain military structure, men inevitably carry this attitude over to their dealings with women.

Romantic involvements between nurses and American men in Vietnam were unavoidable. War tends to link love and youth and passion.[4] When life is reduced to the basic element of staying alive, as it is in war, a person is freed from the inhibitions and restrictions that mark the structured, civilized world. There is exhilaration in this freedom, not unlike the exhilaration of love. Combine the youth of the war participants, freed from societal constraints, with the happiness of having survived another day, and you come to understand why men and women normally absorbed by other concerns found themselves caught up in trysts.

For some, love and romantic involvement was merely an opportunity for sex. There were no long-term commitments or thought of living "happily ever after." Time alone with a man was time to escape from all the destruction and time to receive affection rather than give it. This behavior seemed improper to some people, especially those nurses raised in strict moral environments. But these women came to understand why some of their friends got entangled with men. They realized that preoccupation with men and sex was a form of compensation for all the suffering. Frequently an unguarded moment alone with a man served to preserve a woman's sanity. Without affection and sex, their spirits would be much slower in recuperating from the emotional wounds of their work.

There were plenty of men to choose from and a woman did not have to be gorgeous to attract the attention of many men. Physical looks had little to do with it. Plain people suddenly looked like beauties to love-starved soldiers. An American nurse seemed like the ideal women in Vietnam. She looked, smelled, and acted like home.

Learning to respond to so many men and meeting their own needs for intimacy required a revision in the value system most nurses learned as children. They grew up understanding that they would fall in love and have sex only with the man they would marry. In Vietnam this value system changed. Women learned that love and sex were not always synonymous.

"Territorial bachelors" often taught the nurses about uncommitted sex. This phrase was invented to describe a man, usually an officer, who removed his wedding ring on arrival in Vietnam and kept his marital status hidden until he returned stateside. After a few weeks overseas, the women learned to check the grapevine to seen if their dates were territorial bachelors. Most nurses avoided these men. A few preferred married men because it was easier to be emotionally distant from a man they knew they could never see again. "You had to realize," said one nurse, "that everything in Vietnam was artificial. Everything was transient. You had to learn to put your own needs first to maintain your integrity."

None of the nurses interviewed admitted to promiscuity. Most had one relationship or were serially monogamous during the year in Vietnam. No one apologized for her behavior. Just as they felt no remorse for drinking or other off-duty behavior in Vietnam, these women viewed their personal involvements as acceptable for the time and the place.

Not all nurses adjusted their value systems to the war. There were victims in this changed moral world. One army nurse talked about a friend who got pregnant during a casual sexual encounter and was immediately sent home and discharged from the service. "She put her baby up for adoption and I think of her and that child as war casualties." Other women spoke of two nurses, stationed at different military hospitals, who committed suicide in Vietnam. The reasons for their suicides were not clear, but painful relationships with men were suspected. (Reports of these suicides were not found in official documents.)

Other nurses fell in love. Their attachments were different from the arbitrary wartime romance. Six nurses married men they met in Vietnam. Four couples are still together, and as one women said, "I can not imagine life without him. We understand each other the way few people could." The war put a special imprint on these marriages—a mark of poignancy and sweetness of having survived the war and finding a permanent good among the carnage.

Regardless of how they acted or were affected in Vietnam, the nurses were reluctant to talk about their personal liaisons with men. They were afraid people would not understand why the rules of behavior changed in Vietnam. They also felt that too much emphasis would be placed on this aspect of their wartime tours, thereby trivializing the rest of their experiences. The main reason for their hesitancy was their fear of confirming the long-held myth that women in the military possess a lower moral standard than civilian women.

Rumors of unscrupulous behavior in military women abound. The sources for these myths are not clear but, beginning with the

Revolutionary War when women fought, nursed, and provided domestic services like cooking for the Continental Army, stories about the motives of women serving with so many men inevitably involved sexual behavior.[5] Jean Holm, a retired air force major general who chronicled women's history in the American military, addressed the image: "The record shows that, contrary to the rumors circulated about military women, neither homosexuality or promiscuity were serious problems. The incidence was probably much less than in the general female population."[6]

In "M*A*S*H," one of the most popular television series ever made, actresses portrayed nurses in the Korean War as giggling, mindless females who were the sexual mascots of physicians and other male officers.[7] Such characterizations changed during the later years of the show but those early images stuck. It was not unusual for a nurse back from the war to be asked if Vietnam was really like this television show. Civilians wanted to hear about the wild parties, not about the suffering.

Nurses more experienced with wartime life taught the newcomers to put everything in context. What was acceptable in Vietnam may not be acceptable in the "real world" (a term used to describe life in the United States). Nurses who did not adapt or who brought the coping behavior they had used in Vietnam home had a difficult time dealing with life after the war.

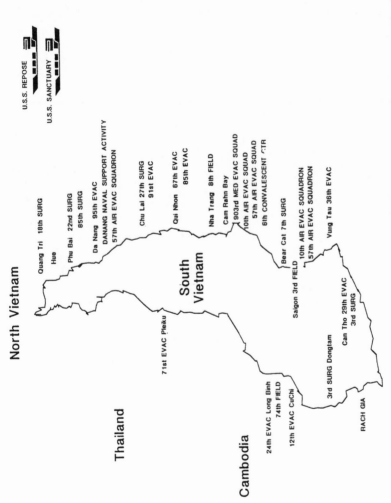

Figure 1: Locations of military facilities where nurses in the study were stationed. Drawing by Mark Papianni, 1989.

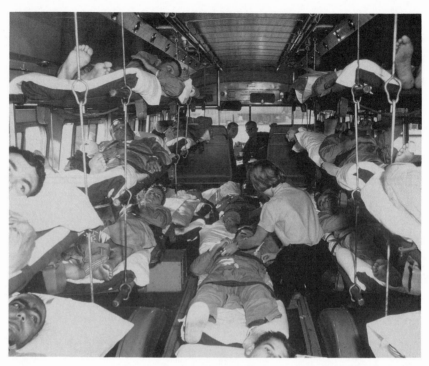

Figure 2: February 1968, Tan Son Nhut AFB, South Vietnam. 2nd Lt. Patricia Hines, USAF, NC 21st Casualty Staging Flight, checks the safety belts of patients aboard an ambulance bus taking wounded servicemen to an aircraft for evacuation to Japan. Source: Official U.S. Air Force Photo, DOD Still Media Records Center

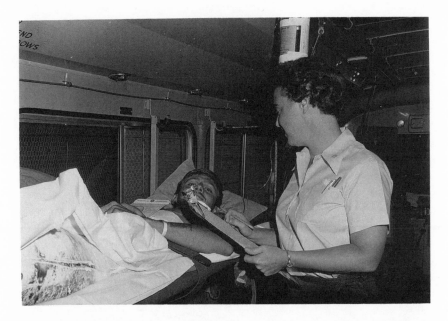

Figure 3: 7 August 1969, Da Nang AFB, South Vietnam. Maj. Dorothy E. Devaney, USAF, NC 22nd Casualty Staging Flight, chats with navy corpsman Vaughn R. Allen aboard an ambulance. Source: Official U.S. Air Force Photo, DOD, Still Media Records Center

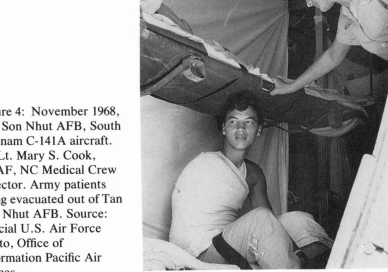

Figure 4: November 1968, Tan Son Nhut AFB, South Vietnam C-141A aircraft. 1st Lt. Mary S. Cook, USAF, NC Medical Crew Director. Army patients being evacuated out of Tan Son Nhut AFB. Source: Official U.S. Air Force Photo, Office of Information Pacific Air Forces

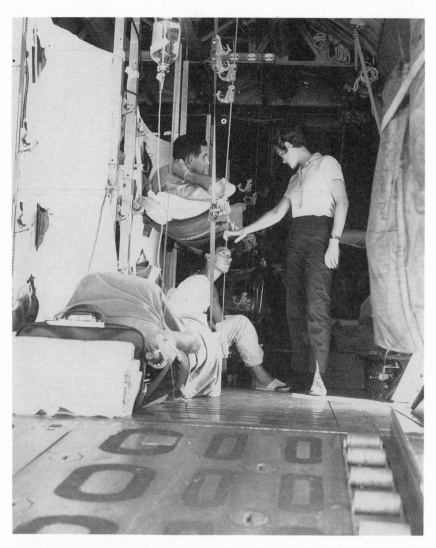

Figure 5: November 1968, Tan Son Nhut AFB, South Vietnam, C-141A aircraft. 1st Lt. Mary S. Cook, USAF, NC Medical Crew Director. Army patients being evacuated out of Tan Son Nhut AFB. Source: Official U.S. Air Force Photo, Office of Information, Pacific Air Forces

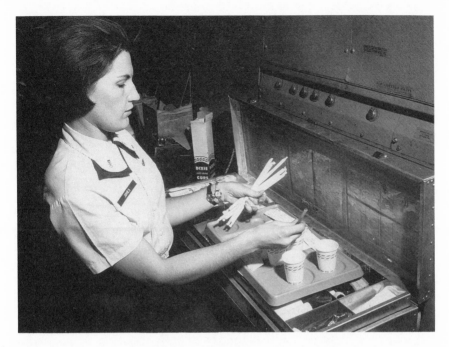

Figure 6: February 1968. 1st Lt. Francis P. Jones, USAF, NC 57th Aero-medical Evacuation Squadron, prepares medications aboard a USAF C-141 aircraft evacuating wounded servicemen from Vietnam to Japan. Source: Official U.S. Air Force Photo, DOD Still Media Records Center

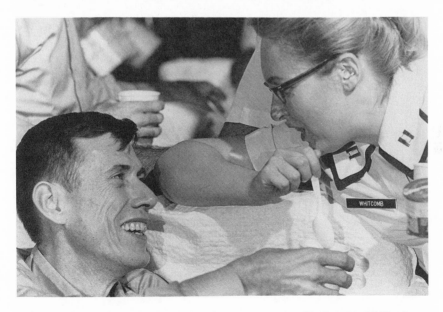

Figure 7: 18 February 1973, aboard a C-141 en route to Clark AFB, Philippines. Capt. E. J. Whitcomb, USAF, NC, talking with newly released P.O.W. Major Joseph Abbot, USAF during "Operation Homecoming." Source: Official U.S. Air Force Photo, DOD Still Media Records Center.

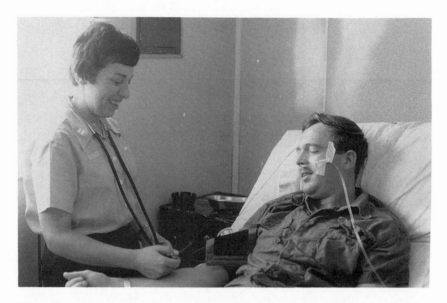

Figure 8: 1969, Tuy Hoa AFB, South Vietnam. Capt. Joann P. Quirrion, USAF, NC the first female nurse assigned to the 31st USAF Dispensary, examines Sgt. Peter N. Owren of the 31st Security Police Squadron. Source: Official U.S. Air Force Photo, DOD, Still Media Records Center

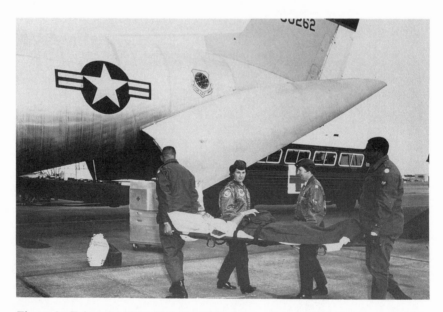

Figure 9: February 1968, Yokota AFB, Japan. A wounded American service-man is carried to a waiting ambulance after being evacuated from Vietnam aboard a U.S. Air Force C-141 aircraft. Source: Official U.S. Air Force Photo, DOD Still Media Records Center

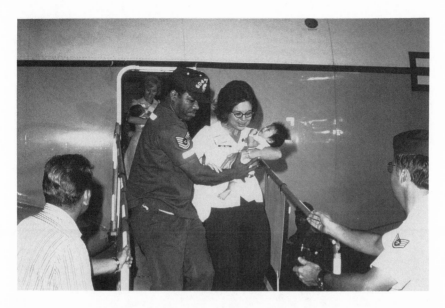

Figure 10: April 1975, C-141 transport plane. An Air Force flight nurse exits a C-141 with a Vietnamese baby during "Operation Babylift" at Clark AFB, Philippines. "Operation Babylift" evacuated children—mostly orphans—from Vietnam prior to the fall of Saigon. Source: Official U.S. Air Force Photo, DOD Still Media Records Center

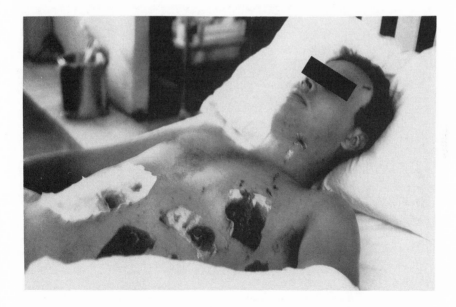

Figure 11: 1969 or 1970, 3rd Field Hospital, Saigon, South Vietnam. Unknown patient with shrapnel wounds. Source: Martha Mosley

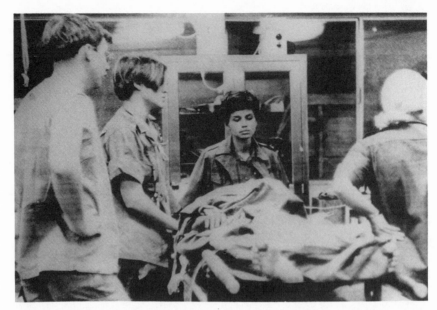

Figure 12: Late 1969, Triage, 71st Evacuation Hospital, South Vietnam. Army medical team working on a massive head trauma patient in triage area. Source: Marra Peche

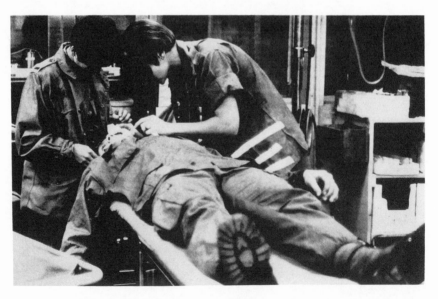

Figure 13: October 1969, 71st Evacuation Hospital, South Vietnam. Two Army nurses cleaning and suturing facial cuts in triage area. Source: Marra Peche

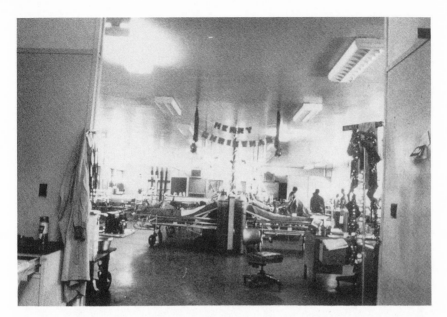

Figure 14: December 1969, 71st Evacuation Hospital, Pleiku, South Vietnam. View as one leaves the operating room and comes to the recovery room (left)/ intensive care unit (right). Source: Marra Peche

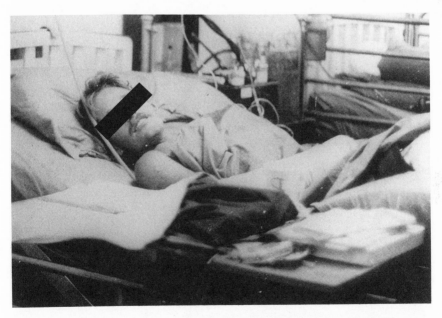

Figure 15: November 1969, 71st Evacuation Hospital, Pleiku, South Vietnam. A wounded patient in the intensive care unit. An Army nurse heard he died during air evacuation to Japan. Source: Marra Peche

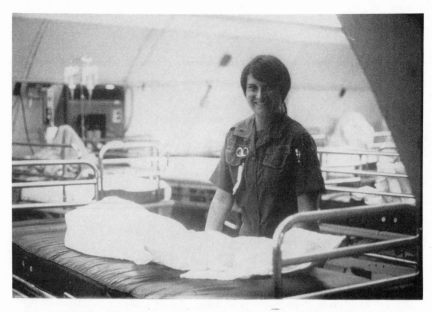

Figure 16: 1969, 67th Evacuation Hospital, Qui Nhon, South Vietnam. 1st Lt. Barbara O'Connor, USA, NC making up a recovery room bed. Source: Lt. Col. Mary Jo Rice

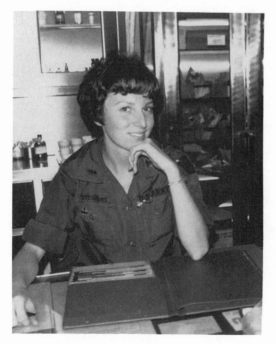

Figure 17: September or October 1970, 12th Evacuation Hospital, Cu Chi, South Vietnam. 1st Lt. Janice Stewart, USA, NC at the nurses' desk on postoperative surgical ward. Source: Janice Stewart

Figure 18: 18 November 1969, 71st Evacuation Hospital, Pleiku, South Vietnam. Lt. Marra Peche, USA, NC on her 25th birthday. Source: Marra Peche

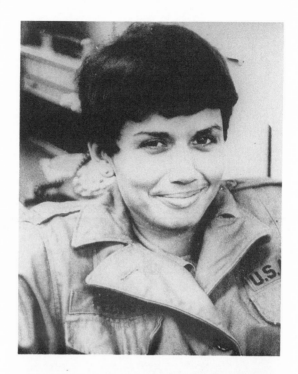

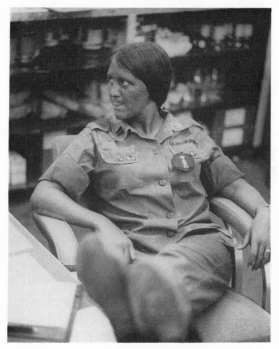

Figure 19: March 1970, 67th Evacuation Hospital, Qui Nhon, South Vietnam. Capt. Mary Jo Rice, USA, NC in the intensive care unit nurses station. Source: Lt. Col. Mary Jo Rice

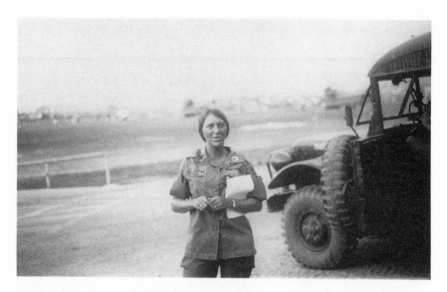

Figure 20: March 1970, 67th Evacuation Hospital, Qui Nhon, South Vietnam. Capt. Mary Jo Rice, USA, NC outside triage near the dustoff helicopter pad in the background. Source: Lt. Col. Mary Jo Rice

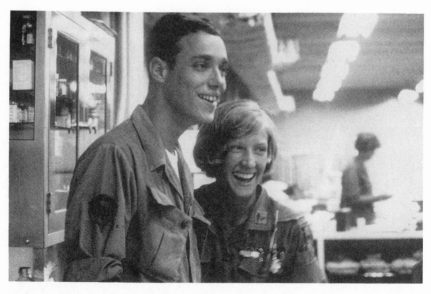

Figure 21: 1969, 67th Evacuation Hospital, Qui Nhon, South Vietnam. 1st Lt. Pamela Years, USA, NC and Sp.5. Max Slifer, 91C in the intensive care unit. Source: Lt. Col. Mary Jo Rice

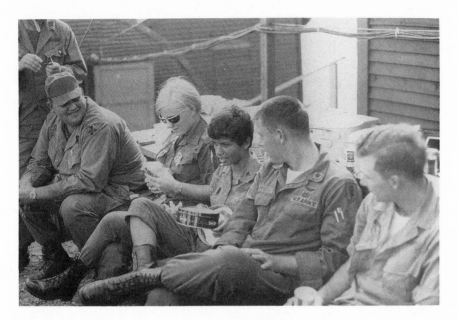

Figure 22: Christmas 1969, Top of Dragon Mountain, II Corps, Vietnam. A farewell to Lt. Marra Peche, USA, NC (holding tin) from close friends. Source: Marra Peche

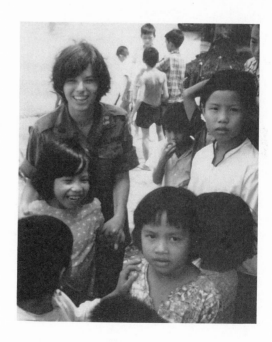

Figure 23: July, 1970, Can Tho, South Vietnam. Lt. Nancy Spears, USA, NC with children in Can Tho South Vietnam. Source: Nancy Spears

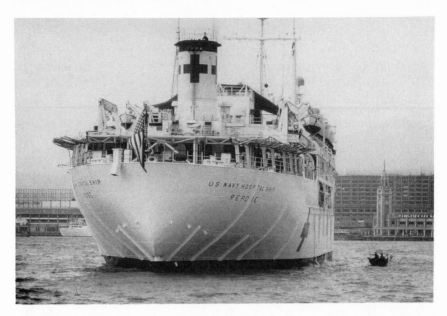

Figure 24: December 1966, Hong Kong Harbor. USS *Repose*-AH-16, as viewed from starboard quarter—on a port call. Source: Capt. Mary Anne Gallagher Ibach USN, NCR

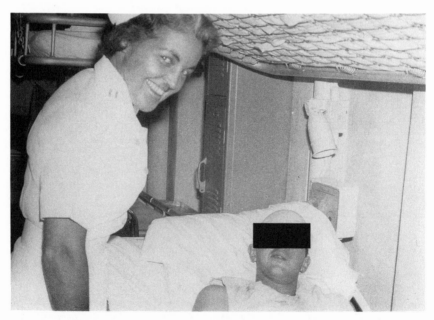

Figure 25: May 1967, USS *Repose* AH-16. Lt. Majorie Thompson USN, NC tends to neurosurgical patient on Ward C-6. Source: Capt. Mary Anne Gallagher Ibach USN, NCR

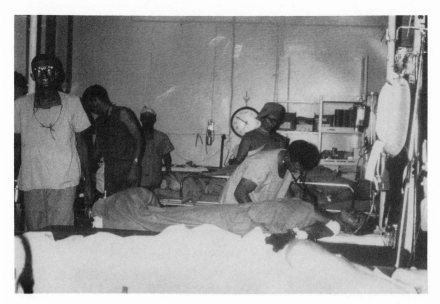

Figure 26: September 1967, USS *Repose*-AH-16, recovery room staging area—pre- and post-anesthesia. Lt. Sandra Jenks USN, NC (standing to right of clock) and recovery room team at work. Source: Capt. Mary Anne Gallagher Ibach USN, NCR

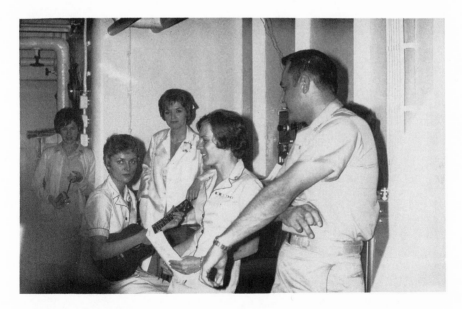

Figure 27: March 1967, wardroom—USS *Repose* AH-16. St. Patrick's Day sing-along. From left Lt. Fran Tomlinson, USN, NC Lt. JG. Roberta Grace USN, NC (with guitar), Lt. Dorothy Leonard USN, NC, Lt. JG. Judy Whitman USN, NC with ship's officer listening in. Source: Capt. Mary Anne Gallagher Ibach USN, NCR

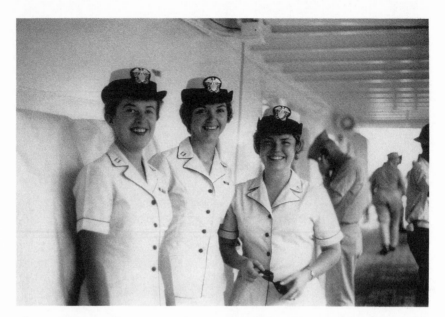

Figure 28: December 1966, USS *Repose* AH-16. Navy nurses on deck. From left Lt. Mary Quinlan, USN, NC Lt. Dorothy Leonard, USN, NC and Lt. JG. Mary Anne Gallagher. USN, NC. Source: Capt. Mary Anne Gallagher Ibach USN, NCR

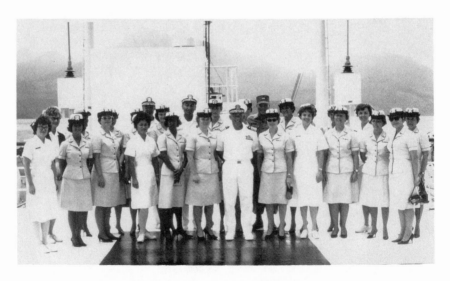

Figure 29: May 1967, USS *Repose* AH-16. Visiting navy and marine corps flag officers with ship's commanding officer and staff nurses on the flying bridge. Source: Capt. Mary Anne Gallagher Ibach USN, NCR

7

Different Experiences in the Army, Navy, and Air Force Nurse Corps

All military nurses experienced certain strains and rewards in Vietnam. Every nurse knew the stress of caring for young patients freshly injured in combat. Every woman learned to adjust to the confinement of ships or military bases. Most nurses enjoyed the special camaraderie that developed among Americans overseas. Regardless of where or when they served in the war, the nurses felt that their skills were appreciated and their judgments about patient care were respected.

There were two factors, however, that colored the nurses' experiences in the war and resulted in different wartime memories. The first factor was the branch of service in which the women served: air force nurses who worked on aircraft had different experiences in Vietnam from navy nurses who worked on hospital ships or army nurses who worked in hospitals throughout South Vietnam. The second factor involved the year the nurse served in Vietnam. This factor is discussed in the next chapter.

The army nurses were land based in Vietnam.[1] The Army nurses in this study worked in three types of medical facilities. The smallest were surgical hospitals like the third Surgical Hospital in Dong Tam, with twenty-four beds in the receiving ward and twenty-four in the main ward. Specialized cases, such as patients with severe kidney injuries or neurologic damage, could not be handled at these small units; these men were sent to larger army evacuation or field hospitals.

Many of these patients went to the ninety-first Evacuation Hospital in Chu Lai, which had three hundred fifty beds. Nurses at evacuation hospitals worked with battle casualties, men with medical illnesses, and civilians. Patients did not usually stay long at the evacuation hospitals: within five days, most men were shipped back to their fighting units or transferred for further care to a rehabilitation hospital in Vietnam or to a hospital in Japan, Guam, Okinawa, the Philippines, Thailand, or the United States.

Field hospitals and convalescent centers, the third type of army facility, were very similar to medical centers back home. Patients there could receive specialized treatment, such as kidney dialysis, and large numbers of patients could be treated. During the 1968 Tet Offensive, the sixth Convalescent Center at Cam Ranh Bay housed fifteen hundred patients in various stages of recuperation. Between four hundred and five hundred of these men were recuperating from hepatitis. Others were recovering from malaria, hookworm, and various tropical illnesses. Still others were surgical combat cases waiting to return to duty.

A rehabilitation battalion at the sixth Convalescent helped recondition soldiers waiting to go back to their units. Every morning, the nurses watched dozens of men jogging around the compound with beautiful Cam Ranh Bay in the background and were reminded of hospitals back home. Only the patients' limps, slightly jaundiced facial color, and thin red suture lines on their arms, legs, and necks indicated they were not stateside.

Living conditions for the army nurses varied. Quarters for the nurses at the ninety-fifth Evacuation Hospital in Da Nang represented living standards at their most basic level. In 1968, sixteen women shared a large tent. The operating room nurses slept in bunks in the back of the tent; the nurses who worked on the wards lived in the front. Clothes were stored in boxes that the enlisted men had made for the nurses. Tentmates learned to be civil to each other at five A.M. and they also learned to sleep through anything—monsoon rain, battle noise, and calls at any hour.

Most army nurses lived in Quonset huts or small buildings, referred to as the "hooches." In Vung Tau, an old resort town on the seacoast, the nurses lived in an old French villa, but any visions of gracious gardens and elegant European architecture this might conjure up would be inaccurate. "It really was an old house," said a nurse who lived at the villa and worked at the thirty-sixth Evacuation Hospital.

Some army nurses had small private rooms. Others shared living quarters. No matter where they lived or in what type of hooch, they all tried to make their rooms comfortable. They used mirrors, stereos, and curtains. Pictures of these interiors showed rooms remarkably like college dormitories.

Sometimes, however, the rooms were not safe. At the seventy-first Evacuation Hospital in Pleiku, flying shrapnel and glass from enemy attacks damaged the nurses' quarters. The force of a typhoon wind from the South China Sea blew off the roof of the nurses' quarters, at the ninety-first Evacuation Hospital in Chu Lai and destroyed all their possessions.

Army nurses lived in Vietnam for twelve months and became more familiar with the people, the countryside, and the long war than the navy or air force nurses, who spent less time on land. Living in the country, they discovered the irony of Vietnam. They saw the countryside pockmarked by mortars and bomb blasts juxtaposed against the beaches and ocean views as beautiful as any vacation resort back home. One army nurse remembered Vietnam in a monochrome of green—the cars, the military buildings, and the clothes.

Life in Vietnam was full of contradictions. The nurses at the ninety-fifth Evacuation Hospital lived in tents, but they had maids to make their bunk beds. They sat in their tents and drank champagne—out of paper cups.

The South Vietnamese not only tolerated the presence of the Americans, they tolerated the enemy as well. The North Vietnamese, Viet Cong, Americans, and South Vietnamese moved and fought in every province.

No where was this strange, and complicated war more apparent then in Vung Tau, the old French resort town located on the ocean. Its miles of beach, open food markets, and Continental restaurants served as a respite from fighting—for both sides. Both the Viet Cong and the Americans used Vung Tau as a "rest and recuperation" center for soldiers needing a break from the war. Army nurses who worked at the thirty-sixth Evacuation Hospital remembered a special set of curfew rules. One nurse explained, "There was a certain line you weren't suppose to cross and a certain time you weren't supposed to be in town. People said that was when they [the Viet Cong] came into town to do their shopping." She laughed at this arrangement.

Army nurses watched symbols of moral strength, military strength, and American culture crumble in the war. The nurses at the twenty-seventh Surgical Hospital saw a priest shot in the abdomen while he said Mass outdoors one spring Sunday. He later died.

During a mass casualty situation at the seventy-first Evacuation Hospital, a nurse looked up from her work with a patient to see a general's aide standing in the middle of the bustling intensive care unit. She asked him what he wanted. He told her he was inspecting the unit to see what was going on. He did not want the general to get upset when he came in to award the patients their Purple Hearts. The nurse reacted with outrage. "I wanted to scream, if you know what I mean. Here are all these brave wounded and dying young men. I told him the general should come down here and get upset." The general never arrived. One of the physicians gave the patients in the intensive care unit their medals.

At another evacuation hospital, a general came to give a Purple Heart to a patient but he arrived too late. The patient died before the ceremony. The army nurse who witnessed the episode was as outraged as her colleague in Pleiku. "This young boy [soldier] died and right afterwards a general pinned a Purple Heart on him. I refused to stand up when the general came in.

Frankly, I was crying and I told him he was a little late with his damn Purple Heart. The general said he understood the stress we were under and he just turned around and left. I still can't believe I did that.''

Both nurses' anger mixed with the realization that they were powerless to stop the dying. After these incidents, both women turned their energies and interest away from the war. For them, the fighting became immoral. They worked only to send their young patients home.

Army nurses in Cu Chi watched the very symbol of American womanhood—Miss America—let them down. The beauty queen was scheduled to visit this large evacuation hospital and lift the spirits of the troops. A nurse who worked at the hospital remembered,

The guys [patients] were so excited. They had something to look forward to. The day of her visit everyone got up early to help the patients shave and get ready. Well, she arrived, but we didn't see her. Apparently she broke out in a heat rash and snubbed the boys. She never came to the hospital. They were so disappointed. We were furious. I figured I was better than her dressed up in my fatigues than she was in her sexy dress.[2]

The nurses had learned firsthand the shallowness of the symbols that were supposed to support the troops and the war effort; they saw that Vietnam emphasized the best and the worst in human behavior. They would be quick to point out they did not suffer the terror of battle or the discomfort of jungle living. But they clearly viewed the human costs of war by spending twelve months caring for the casualties of battle. They saw the moral disintegration and the long-term physical consequences. The nurses knew better than military commanders that a lifetime of pain and disability was waiting for some men after Vietnam.

Additionally, contrary to the long-held myth that nurses in war zones were safe, twenty-four of the fifty nurses recalled being exposed to enemy fire three or more times during their tours.[3] The myth had developed out of the public's perception that the hospitals were far away from the fighting; they believed the nurses would never have to fear for their lives. But in Vietnam, there were no front lines and no safe areas. The guerrilla nature of the war made every place and everyone vulnerable to attack.

The most frequent dangers to army and other land-based nurses were enemy rockets, mortars, and artillery. Helicopter landing pads, which had large, painted markings, were targets of enemy fire. If they were destroyed, wounded patients could not be brought in from the battlefield. Some hospitals seemed more vulnerable than others. For example, nurses at the twenty-second Surgical Hospital in Phu Bai spent five months from February to June 1968 confined to their compound because of frequent enemy attacks. During the Tet Offensive of 1968, a nurse who worked at the twenty-seventh Surgical Hospital in Chu Lai remembered incoming mortars and rockets going over the hospital every night for weeks on end.

Enemy attacks occurred in unexpected places like Saigon, South Vietnam's capital city, and Cam Ranh Bay. At the third Field Hospital in Saigon, military guards found maids smuggling eighty pounds of explosive plastique into the nurses' quarters. The maids carried enough plastique to make a bomb that could have leveled the nurses' building. In Cam Ranh Bay, sapper (terrorist) squads swam in from the sea, blew down a water tower, machine gunned the doctors' quarters, and shot some of the ambulatory patients as they ran for cover. No one was safe.

At the Naval Support Activity (NSA) Da Nang, the only naval hospital facility on land in Vietnam, enemy rounds aimed at the Marine Air Group frequently fell short and landed in the hospital compound. A nurse who worked at NSA Da Nang described an attack: "One night it was pretty bad. I didn't think I was going to be wounded or die but it was frightening. We lost half a ward. They blew up the urology clinic and they blew in the door of the ICU [intensive care unit]. Patients got rewounded. A corpsman lost a eye. We used to get showered with shrapnel in the wards."[4]

Everyone felt so vulnerable. People had no weapons to defend themselves and there was no underground shelter to run for protection. Patients with combat experience knew the sound of incoming mortars. They knew they could be killed lying helpless in bed, here in the one place in Vietnam people wanted to feel safe. Nurses remember patients screaming for their weapons or crying out in fear and anger as the rockets hit, "My god, this is a hospital!"

When the alert sirens went off, nurses on duty knew what to do. Each hospital ward had a shelf with helmets and flak jackets. After putting them on, the nurses helped prepare patients. Men crawled or were lifted off their beds and stretchers and placed on the floor. The women put helmets on their patients and placed flak jackets over their bodies. Some nurses had to disconnect orthopedic traction to move men. Critically ill patients who could not be moved were left in their beds but covered with mattresses to protect them from dust and flying glass and shrapnel

Nursing care continued during the attacks. Emergency generators provided electricity for life-support equipment such as respirators while the rest of hospital remained in darkness. Nurses worked with flashlights, occasionally crawling around on their hands and knees to check and to reassure their patients.

Even off-duty women were in dangerous situations. One nurse remembered being shot at while driving to a village to administer vaccines. Another woman recalled a face to face encounter with the enemy. She said, "I agreed to go with this guy dancing at a camp across town. I guess it was about a mile away. I put on my yellow dress and we got in a jeep. As we were rounding a curve, this man in black pajamas [the uniform of the Viet Cong] is standing right in front of us. He lifted his rifle and looked me right in the eye. I thought I was dead, but he put the rifle down and we drove on." She will never know why he did not pull the trigger, but her sense of invincibility disappeared that night.

The near presence of death and the prospect of meeting it at the next moment moved the nurses in curious ways. Dreamers became realists. The frightened found courage. Before going to Vietnam, most nurses had been unconcerned about their personal safety. The war was the first time in their lives they had to face their own mortality. As one nurse summed up the general reaction to this personal danger, "You grow up fast."

There was also a sense of exhilaration and a sense of excitement. Nurses at the twelfth Evacuation Hospital in Cu Chi would climb on the roof of a latrine and watch the tracers and the helicopter firefights right outside the compound wire. Nurses at Da Nang remember drinking scotch and water in the officers' club while watching mortars explode nearby. There was noise and color. They knew they were witnesses to a great human drama. It was not until the next hours or day, when the casualties arrived, that reality returned and they remembered what such excitement cost.

By contrast, the experience of the navy nurses in this study in the Vietnam War took place on the South China Sea. The three navy nurses stationed at the Da Nang Navy Support Hospital and the one assigned to Rach Gia, a French provincial hospital, had wartime experiences that more closely resembled those of the army nurses than those of their colleagues on the hospital ships.

The navy nurses who worked on either the USS *Repose* or the USS *Sanctuary* spent ninety days "on-line"—the military term for active service in the war zone. The ships sailed off the coast of Vietnam, receiving and caring for patients wounded in battle or suffering from tropical diseases. During quiet times, helicopter pilots brought children to the ships for elective surgeries to repair congenital anomalies like cleft lips.

The amount of time the hospital ships and their crews spend on-line was significant because carriers, destroyers, and other ships in "the Gray Navy" were on-line for only thirty days, and this length of time was considered a hardship. "We stayed on-line three times the length of the gray ships," recalled a Navy commander. "It wasn't easy, but we were proud that we had more resilience than the fighting ships." At one point during intense fighting, the USS *Sanctuary* was on-line for 120 days. There were too many casualties for the crew to leave.

In 1966, during its early service in the war, the USS *Repose* used to drop anchor off Da Nang. However, after one episode when Viet Cong divers tried to mine the ship's anchor, commanding officers decided it was safer to remain at sea and make home port a naval base far from the war. As a result, both hospital ships cruised in slow figure eight patterns on the South China Sea.

Every three months, the ships went to the huge naval base at Subic Bay in the Philippines for repairs and installation of new equipment. Everyone looked forward to the ten days spent in dry dock because it gave them an opportunity to shop, eat in restaurants, sleep in "real" beds, and take baths. Subic Bay was their refuge from the war.

Women were a minority on board ship—some thirty nurses versus a male crew of several hundred men. Living space was at a premium and quarters were cramped. A picture of the nurses' living quarters shows uniforms hanging on the back of a door and bunk beds in a room that looks like a small closet. Yet no one complained about the close quarters. The nurses knew that few women in the navy at that time had the opportunity to experience shipboard life as they did.

Shipboard areas where nurses and other personnel could socialize were strictly designated. The nurses had their own sun deck that was off limits to male personnel. Mixed groups congregated in the officers' mess to eat and to relax or on the ship's deck to look at the sea and the sunsets. Sometimes they would watch nearby battles that looked like fireworks over a lake on the Fourth of July. Then the helicopters would land with their casualties and reality would return.

It was a regimented life both at work and off-duty. To deal with the lifestyles and work stresses, navy men and women developed close social relationships. There was a different dynamic to life aboard ship, a bonding born of isolation and confinement. "We became a big family, which made it much easier to be at sea for so long," said a nurse from the USS *Sanctuary*.

To deal with shipboard life, the nurses also tried to maintain a sense of home. Medical personnel followed the patterns of navy life stateside. The nurses wore the traditional white dresses and caps at work and were expected to be in military uniform at other times. Civilian clothes were allowed only on the sun deck. The rules of social conduct gave their lives structure in a confined, often tense environment.

The navy nurses' workplace was very different from that of stateside hospitals. All the equipment and machines were tied down to guard against pitching and rolling in heavy seas. Patients were stacked in three tiers of beds or racks that hung from the ceiling by chains. A nurse who spent a year working on the USS *Repose* remembered, "You had to tie the suction machines down so they wouldn't roll all over the place. We had Stryker frames tied from one pole to other. I often wondered what the patients on those frames felt like, being turned back to stomach when the ship was rolling side to side.''[5]

Nurses also had to adjust to life at sea. It often took several weeks and several doses of Dramamine before the women got their sea legs. No sailor—and all navy personnel consider themselves sailors—wanted to admit to seasickness.

The nurses sometimes listened to ''Hanoi Hannah''—the Vietnam War's equivalent to World War II's ''Tokyo Rose,'' on the radio. Hannah was a well-known North Vietnamese radio announcer and propaganda specialist who reported U.S. military movements and encouraged Americans to surrender before their ''inevitable defeat.'' Nurses remember one particular broadcast when Hannah announced, ''Well, *Repose,* you are going to be blown out of the water on September 16th.'' They thought the threat was hollow, but when the day arrived, there was a general uneasiness on the ship.

Other instances of danger were more real. One day, the USS *Sanctuary* lost all power at sea and the machines that kept the patients alive stopped working. A nurse remembers people voluntarily coming to the intensive care unit to give oxygen manually to patients. No one died during that hour-long blackout.

There also was the environmental stress of riding out a typhoon at sea. Hospital ships were top heavy, so the rolls during a storm were severe. Nurses who slept on top bunks spent stormy nights sleeping on the floor for fear they would fall out during a heavy sea swell. Five nurses remembered a particular typhoon that hit a ship while it was in the Philippines. ''One time the ship rolled to its side and hesitated,'' said one of these women who turned her hand to illustrate the ship's movement in the storm. ''Just for a second you didn't know which way it would go.'' She moved her hand upside down and then upright to illustrate the options. (The ship remained up.) Meanwhile, patients below deck felt helpless with their injuries; many feared drowning and had to be reassured.

On one occasion the USS *Repose,* filled with patients, collided with an oil tanker during refueling. The collision left the deck awash with highly volatile fuel and a hole in the ship just above the water line. No one was hurt and crewmen repaired the ship.

The USS *Forrestal,* an aircraft carrier stationed off Vietnam, was not so lucky. In 1967, a plane blew up on the carrier's deck, setting off a series of explosions and fires down several decks of the ship. A distress call went out for help with the fire and for a hospital ship. The navy nurses on the ship that responded remember this episode as the most stressful experience of the war. As they came alongside the wounded ship, the nurses of the USS *Repose* watched the fires and heard the shouts of the men.

It was the dead of night and all you could see were red lights and the flames. All you could hear was the whirl of helicopters and the banging of men trapped below deck. We expected to admit casualties but what we got were bodies. Actually, we received twelve live casualties and seventy to ninety bodies and parts of bodies. The casualties were in terrible shape. Some of the men had been blown off the deck into the water so they were burned and they had multiple fractures. Our morgue did not have enough room. By ten P.M. we dumped the food out of our freezers to hold all the bodies. I remember opening a bag and finding a torso with a gold oak leaf. I was probably looking at a young Lieutenant commander aviator. The corpsmen started to cry. All night long we worked. We expected to help people, but we became a morgue. Our whole ship was somber.

The next morning there was a beautiful blue sky. We had a memorial Mass. The [USS] *Forrestal* headed to the Philippines for repair. She was listing as she steamed away. Her crewmen were standing on deck: a sailor, a marine, a sailor, a marine—all the way around the flight deck in salute to those men who died the night before. We went to Da Nang and stood at attention as they off-loaded the bodies from our ship. When I think about it today I can still smell the fire and see the bodies.

Not all air force nurses were assigned to flight duty throughout the war; approximately 150 nurses worked in fixed (ground) hospital facilities in Vietnam and Thailand. Air force nurse corps officers had had both military and nursing experience prior to their overseas duty. Initial Active Duty nurses (individuals in their first three-year military tour) were not assigned to Southeast Asia.[6]

The air force nurses in this study spent most of their time in aircraft ferrying patients to hospitals within Vietnam or to Japan and the United States.[7] Those nurses who flew medical evacuation "in-country" spent a year, like the army nurses, living and working in South Vietnam. Home base for these nurses was at one of the three major air fields: Da Nang Airport, Cam Ranh Bay Airport, and Tan Son Nhut Airport in Saigon. These nurses, unlike their army counterparts, came to know the whole countryside rather than just one area. They landed everywhere from the central highlands near Pleiku in the north to the Mekong Delta in the southern end of the country.

A typical day involved ten to fourteen landings at various airfields. To talk to one of these nurses is to hear a very different description of Vietnam. They knew where to buy the best fresh fruit, and they knew about the prison island off South Vietnam where enemy prisoners lived in cages. They knew the stores that sold the best jade jewelry, and they knew which were the most friendly or most antagonistic South Vietnamese villages and cities.

During their first weeks in Vietnam, air force nurses spent time in flight training with experienced instructors and learned about the laws of physics and the location of fuel tanks on aircraft. The patients under their care were exposed to conditions known as "the stresses of flight." As aircraft climbed into the atmosphere, the barometric pressure and humidity level in the planes decreased. (Barometric pressure is the term used to describe the amount of tension exerted on gases in the atmosphere.)[8]

Military aircraft were not as pressurized as commercial planes so the amount of oxygen available decreased rapidly on medical evacuation flights. Patients with chest traumas, head injuries, or any type of bleeding—all disorders that compromised the ability to breathe normally—needed diligent monitoring for signs of hypoxia (lack of oxygen). Some of the signs nurses watched for in these men were increased restlessness, increased breathing and pulse, and a bluish color in the patients' nail beds. Nurses needed to know the location of and how to operate the oxygen masks and cannulas on every aircraft.

As the barometric pressure dropped in the evacuation planes, gases normally found in the human body can and do expand. Soldiers with ear and facial wounds were particularly susceptible to painful sinus injury because gases inside their heads expanded and could not escape. Nurses learned to check vulnerable patients and administer antihistamine drugs to them before takeoff to avoid this airborne complication. Men with abdominal injuries would experience bloated abdomens when gas expanded and got trapped in their bowels. Nurses alleviated this condition by passing a tube down their patients' noses and into their stomachs to deflate the expansion. Another problem occurred when gases located in the bloodstream expanded and newly closed suture lines ruptured. Nurses examined all wounds frequently during flying times and became skilled in tourniquet application and blood transfusions.

The lack of humidity on the aircraft caused sore throats, parched skin, and even dry eyeballs for both patients and crew. These conditions were not only uncomfortable: the low humidity made breathing more difficult by drying out breathing passages and causing rapid evaporation of moisture from the skin. Everyone was vulnerable to dehydration on long flights, so nurses made sure there was plenty to drink. They also checked intravenous lines to make sure unconscious and wounded patients received enough fluid.

As crew members of a flying group, nurses had to know the location of safety equipment and what to do if a crash was imminent or occurred. The women worked in three types of aircraft during their Vietnam tours. Two planes, the C-123s and the C-130s, were propeller cargo planes that had been converted for medical use. There was nothing comfortable about these aircraft, but they were very efficient in the war. Pilots could land them in the dirt on short runways. Pilots easily made the steep forty-five-degree angle climbs and descents (called combat climbs) in sheer terrain or when aircraft were under attack. A third type of aircraft, C-9s, were the only planes specifically built for medical evacuation. These looked like hospitals with suction and oxygen equipment secured in the walls and places to hang intravenous fluid.

Once they had completed their training period in Vietnam, nurses were considered qualified flight personnel. Training was rigorous. Physicians rarely flew air evacuation flights, so nurses assumed responsibility for all patient care decisions.

Early each morning, air force nurses learned the type of plane they would fly that day. They also received an itinerary listing all expected destinations. These lists were flexible because needs quickly changed with new battles or when a patient somewhere needed emergency evacuation. The C-123 and C-130 aircraft often contained cargo during the first flight of the day. Once crewmen unloaded the equipment, three types of patients walked or were carried aboard: those just injured in combat, those with severe injuries requiring a neurosurgeon or other specialist, and those with medical diseases, usually malaria. Work days were long. One nurse said she usually left at five A.M. and returned to Cam Ranh Bay Airport between ten or eleven P.M.

Sunday was the only day the crew did not receive a planned schedule, just answering only emergency calls. These calls seemed to come regularly. Most of the time, flight nurses and their squadrons worked seven days a week. Night missions were rare because of increased enemy activity. Crews answered only urgent calls to transport critically injured Americans.

Other air force nurses spent long hours flying patients from Vietnam to Japan and the United States. These flights began in Vietnam, where nurses "staged" or prepared their patients for the journey out of the war. After landing in Japan, the crew picked up other patients and continued stateside. They then flew back to Vietnam to repeat the circuit. The six-, ten-, or twelve-hour flights to Japan and the United States involved nonstop rounds of monitoring, assessing, and soothing wounded men. Professional responsibility and fatigue were the major stress factors for air force nurses.

These nurses quickly realized they could not dwell on the dangers of flying. If they worried, how would they be able to fly the next day? Emotional discipline became part of their work. The enemy did not distinguish one American aircraft from another.[9] "I can remember a couple of times," said one flight nurse, "when the plane started to move before the doors were closed. We had to get in the air because they were shooting at us."

Another reason the women were not troubled about their personal safety was the example of the patients. One flight nurse who remembered many near crashes in Vietnam said, "You have to understand that I didn't think about things like [personal safety] because the situations I was in are so minimal compared to the situations of the young men there. Why should I worry about an airplane getting shot down when I see some kid with both his legs off? I got to eat hot meals and drink cold drinks. We [her squadron] had refrigerators and electricity. I got to change my clothes, unlike the men.'' After transporting hundreds of wounded men, seeing their wounds, and hearing their stories of combat and jungle living, flight nurses rarely felt the danger of their own work.

8

Factors Associated with the Year the Nurse Served in Vietnam

Year by year, the war ebbed and flowed. The nurses stationed in Vietnam during 1965 at the start of the major U.S. build-up had different experiences from the nurses who served in 1971, when the United States was in a period of de-escalation. Public support and opinion back home directly affected troop morale. Earlier, when civilian support for American objectives and goals in Vietnam was strong, military men and women had accepted the battles and their subsequent casualties as an awful but necessary price to win the war. But later in the war years, everything changed. Widespread vocal public criticism of the war left American military personnel questioning the value of their sacrifices.[1] As moral confusion and a sense of abandonment spread among the forces, nurses began to see patients with drug overdoses, self-inflicted gunshot wounds, and injuries from racial fights.

The American public never questioned the nurses' role in the war. The nurses never suffered the stigma army troops experienced after the My Lai massacre.[2] (In March 1968, a U.S. infantry company slaughtered more than three hundred Vietnamese inhabitants of My Lai village.) Still, these women considered themselves part of the military. Thus, they absorbed and endured the harsh civilian reactions.

Later in the war years, many military draftees and other personnel shared the public antiwar sentiment. Those nurses who felt American involvement in Vietnam was wrong began to view the wounded and the dead with a sense of futility. They were angry at a conflict that claimed lives for a dubious cause.

One navy nurse arrived in Vietnam before most American servicemen. She had been on active duty in the navy nurse corps since the Korean War. She was an experienced operating room nurse, and was committed to a lifelong military career. Single, she had worked around the world in different military facilities. Other navy nurses described her as independent and confident. In 1964, as her tour of duty was ending stateside, she knew her next assignment would be overseas. Nothing, however, in her lengthy nursing experience had prepared her for the directive that ordered her to a small then relatively unknown country in Southeast Asia.

On March 8, 1965, the first American combat troops reached Vietnam. A marine regiment landed to defend the Da Nang airport.[3] That same month, the navy nurse flew to Saigon as part of a tri-service medical team sent to a hospital in Rach Gia, a provincial capital in the Delta region of South Vietnam. Her team consisted of two navy physicians, two navy nurses and a laboratory x-ray technician, an air force nurse-anesthetist, and an army administrative officer in charge of supplies. They went to Vietnam as advisers from the Agency for International Development; they did not have military uniforms or identification tags. Their assignment was to train their Vietnamese counterparts in Western operating room methods.

The group arrived in Vietnam with their own pots and pans. They were even greeted by local politicians. A banner hung across the main street of the local village read: "Welcome U.S. Surgical team." They set to work and quickly integrated themselves into the local scene. They ate native food, but made an occasional trip to Saigon for supplies and a special treat of ice cream. One of the nurses drove a truck around the village. The Americans "adopted" a local orphan and, when they left Vietnam, they gave the mother superior money to send the boy to school.

To the locals, the surgical team must have seemed more like neutral missionaries than military personnel. This neutrality was most evident the day they received a patient from another local hospital. The administrators of this hospital were known to be Viet Cong. The sick man arrived with the message, "Can you help this patient?"

"We had a trusting and reciprocal relationship with the Vietnamese. We were totally accepted by them," she said. Five years later mistrust and antagonism were the rule. But these early advisers were so successful in their mission that aspiring politicians wanted to see their work. The navy nurse remembered the day in 1965 when Richard Nixon, on a fact-finding tour, came for lunch. The future president of the United States was then a New York lawyer.

The year passed quickly. "No one," she said, "felt pressure to come home." In subsequent years, American personnel made calendars with their DEROS (Date of Expected Return from Overseas) clearly and brightly marked. This nurse looks back on her tour with great satisfaction. She would "do it all over again in a minute."

Other women in the study arrived later in 1965 to serve on board the hospital ships or to work at various army facilities like the third Field Hospital in Saigon or the eighty-fifth Evacuation Hospital in Qui Nhon. Air force nurses began flying medical evacuation missions. By December 1965, American troop strength was two hundred thousand men. A year later, the number reached nearly four hundred thousand men.[4]

No one knows the number of female military nurses in Vietnam during any year of the war. It is logical to assume, however, that as the numbers of combat troops increased, so did the numbers of nurses. Most of the nurses in this study, twenty-eight out of fifty women, were in Vietnam during 1967, 1968, and 1969, when troop strength was at its peak.

The nurses who served early in the war, between 1965 and

1967, had a sense of esprit de corps. They felt the support of society back home. "We had a sense of purpose, a sense that we mattered. When I got there it was still okay to be a marine and go off to Vietnam," said a nurse who spent 1966 on board the USS *Repose*. The American military continued to possess the self-assurance they had developed during World War II. Drug problems among the troops were minimal. It was unusual for soldiers to write home about their anger and guilt.[5]

When the pace of work slowed, nurses wrote letters home for their patients. A navy lieutenant recalled enclosing a note in a package she wrapped for a wounded marine. "I wrote to his mother and told her how nice her son was and how proud she should be of him." In return, patients often gave nurses small gifts—unit insignia, a small-size set of Korean fatigues, a poncho liner to keep warm in the monsoon rains. Patients on shore leave from the hospital ships brought the nurses back such gifts as perfume.

The cohesive environment of 1966 and 1967 helped the nurses cope with the professional demands of their work. Here was wartime military nursing as most women imagined it to be—long hours, wounded men, difficult working conditions, but days filled with satisfaction and a sense that they were part of a heritage of care that extended back to previous wars.

In the latter months of 1967, things began to change. The pace of the war and the numbers of casualties increased and American sympathy for the cause began to turn.

Nurses remember the Tet Offensive of 1968 as a time of fierce battles and large numbers of wounded. On January 31, 1968, the start of the lunar new year celebration called "Tet," seventy thousand enemy troops launched an offensive on hundreds of Vietnamese towns and villages and American military installations. The swift attacks surprised the Americans. Fierce battles and terrible casualties followed.[6]

Eight of the nurses interviewed served in Vietnam during this time. One army nurse on the coast of Vietnam at the eighty-fifth Evacuation Hospital in Qui Nhon recalled the intensity of the offensive: "We could actually witness a battle going on in the hills above us. We watched the gunships fire, the assualt, the enemy firing back." Nurses across Qui Nhon at the sixty-seventh Evacuation Hospital adjusted to sleeping under their beds with flak jackets on and helmets nearby. They frequently worked by flashlight during attacks and alerts.

Up the seacoast at Chu Lai, nurses at the twenty-seventh Surgical Hospital received vast numbers of casualties. Closer to Saigon, at an American base named "Bear Cat," commanders thought the base and hospital were going to be overrun. The chief nurse told her staff about the imminent danger, but ordered them not to warn the patients because little could be done for the wounded and sick if the hospital were to be overrun. Everyone spent thirty days under constant alert. The big attack never came.

It was an unnerving time. News of the assault on the American Embassy in Saigon reached the nurses and many feared an enemy victory. Some recalled the nurses who were captured in the Philippines during World War II. According to autobiographies written by two women in this group, sixty-seven army nurse corps and twelve navy nurse corps officers spent thirty-seven months in the Japanese prison camps at Los Baños and Santo Tomás in the Philippines.[7] A similar capture, they thought, could happen again.

Yet there was little time to ponder overall political and military conditions because mass casualty situations occurred with regularity. Marines were wounded in the Battle of Hue. Infantrymen and sailors were hurt fighting in the Mekong Delta. Soldiers and civilians were injured by terrorist attacks in Saigon. The victims kept arriving. "Every ten minutes another helicopter landed with casualties," said a young lieutenant.

Supplies ran short. Nurses kept the one washing machine on the USS *Repose* working twenty-four hours a day so that operating room personnel did not run out of the absorbent bandages that were needed for surgery. Other nurses improvised. At one hospital, there were so many men with chest traumas that nurses used up every bottle in the facility trying to collect the blood that oozed from the wounds. They resorted to using urinary drainage bags to gather the chest serum. In other hospitals, army cots were taken apart and the wooden supports used to splint fractured extremities. When an evacuation hospital ran short of antibiotics, medics went to the Vietnamese ward in the hospital and took what was left of these drugs to use on the Americans. Enlisted men frequently gave blood to bolster the dwindling supplies. (Nurses rarely donated blood because commanders wanted the women to preserve their stamina for work.) They bartered with other hospitals for needed provisions, and flight nurses ferried gear between the various facilities.

Army nurses sent enlisted men out to scrounge equipment. One navy nurse said she never worried about shortages because, "that's what chiefs are for in the navy." These chief petty officers and supply sergeants were streetwise men who found whatever the nurses requested. Sometimes these men borrowed supplies, sometimes they stole them; in true military tradition, they never revealed their sources.

Each January for the remainder of the war, Americans troops became uneasy as the Tet holiday neared. In 1970, nurses remembered being restricted to post for the holiday. Such action proved unnecessary because the enemy never again launched a massive military offensive like the one in 1968.

Back home, meanwhile, the antiwar movement gained momentum as mostly young and draft-age Americans began to questions the worth of fighting and dying in the war. On April 15, 1967, large antiwar demonstrations took place in New York and San Francisco. During the autumn of 1967, fifty young men held a public burning of their draft cards in Boston, Massachusetts. Chicago police attacked and arrested antiwar protesters at the 1968 Democratic National Convention. The first Vietnam Moratorium Day was held on October 15, 1969 when college campuses across the country became the setting for antiwar lectures, guerrilla theater, and protest marches. Large-scale antiwar demonstrations continued through 1970, 1971, and 1972. Four hundred colleges and universities closed during May 1970 as hundreds of thousands of students protested President Nixon's decision to use American troops to invade Cambodia. Four students at Kent State University died during an antiwar demonstration that May when Ohio National Guardsmen fired their rifles to disperse a crowd. The next year, in May 1971, Washington, D.C., police arrested ten thousand protesters during a May Day demonstration.[8]

Slowly, the connection with the past began to disintegrate. Support on the "home front" was something that had been taken for granted, something that was expected. Now, the public shouted slogans, "Hell no, we won't go!" and "Ho, Ho, Ho Chi Minh / NLF is gonna win!" (Ho Chi Minh was the president of North Vietnam, the NLF was the National Liberation Front, an organization of South Vietnam's communists whose members were more commonly referred to as Viet Cong.)[9] American actress Jane Fonda visited Hanoi to show her support for the North Vietnamese. Nurses remember the actress calling Americans troops "dupes and suckers." Fonda and others who opposed American policy in Vietnam viewed the Americans serving in Vietnam as agents of a corrupt American political system.[10]

The antiwar movement angered the nurses. They felt that the Americans protesting the war were turning their backs on the wounded. These nurses saw Fonda's trip to Hanoi as a treasonous act. It was especially unsettling to watch another American woman endorse the same enemy who was causing the death and suffering the nurses saw each day. Reaction against Fonda's action remains strong, perhaps particularly because she is a woman. One former army nurse said, "To this day, I will never see or participate in anything that Jane Fonda has to do with. I will not see her movies or watch her exercise videos. She had *her* campaign; well, this is *my* one woman campaign."

Not all nurses remained unswerving in their support of the war. Still, although some women questioned military strategy, their loyalty to their patients overshadowed their personal political views.

The peace movement and racial strife between blacks and whites back home also combined to bring discord to the ranks in Vietnam. Soldiers, agitated by urban riots and growing black militancy, segregated themselves.[11] The separate racial groups ate, slept, and relaxed together; they would antagonize others outside their own clique.

At one large base on the South China Sea, nurses remembered watching military police disarm all black soldiers because there was fear of bloodshed. In two other incidents, nurses remembered admitting soldiers to hospitals with gunshot wounds and booby trap injuries received in racially motivated fights.

One nurse related an incident that occurred while she was shopping for Christmas presents in Saigon.

I had my money and ID in my breast pocket. These little kids pushed against me. My pocket was open and my money gone. I saw one of the kids, grabbed him, and started screaming "You've got my money, give it back!" The police were across the street watching the whole thing.

These four black soldiers came up and grabbed the kid and asked me what happened. I was crying and told them about the robbery and my money. They [the soldiers] let the kid go. They just walked away. I heard one guy say, "She's not a sister."

I went crazy. I was screaming, "I'm an American!" It was bad enough being robbed of your Christmas money but to have Americans come up and not help me because they were black and I wasn't. They probably couldn't have done anything, but."

She was stunned and furious. Camaraderie was a basic tenet of wartime military life. To her, the incident made a lie of her patriotism and her desire to serve, the reason she had volunteered for duty in Vietnam.

Vietnam was the first time many nurses experienced political and moral conflict. These women had grown up believing in equality for all people. Suddenly, they found themselves serving in a war and in a world no one seemed to understand. One nurse described this conflict: "Your whole world was falling apart. You believed in your work as a nurse but the war seemed so crazy."

Everyone wanted the fighting and the casualties to end. As the years passed, more women felt frustrated with the slow process toward peace. One night in the summer of 1969, a navy nurse was on duty at the hospital in Da Nang the day Neil Armstrong set foot on the moon. The event made her think: Here she was facing a ward of injured young men, and "all I could think was that we had the technology to get to the moon but we couldn't even figure out how to have peace on earth."

An army nurse who worked at the sixty-seventh Evacuation Hospital in Qui Nhon in 1968 and 1969 described a pattern that was followed by many nurses: "I went over [to Vietnam] with very idealistic thoughts that we're here to help these people and save their country. After I was there for three or four months, I came to realize that the Vietnamese didn't really care that we were there or not. All they wanted was to make money off the Americans—to take our aid. I became cynical. I don't think they cared whether the communists took over the country or not."

At some hospitals an effort to bolster sagging morale was undertaken by military commanders who presented lectures on patriotism and politics in the base chapels. But these mandatory sessions had the opposite effect. Returning to a ward full of burned marines and soldiers wounded by grenades, one woman thought the propaganda was just plain silly.

The Vietnamese black market, which flourished and drained essential materials was another source of great irritation because patients suffered from compromised care. It also illustrated to the nurses the indifference of some Vietnamese to their own cause. The seventy-first Evacuation Hospital in Pleiku, for example, was situated in the highlands of South Vietnam, a place of cold nights and rainy days. Army issue poncho liners, sweat shirts, and green wool socks provided some comfort, but in 1971, these supplies never reached the nurses stationed there because they were being sold at the local black market. The women had to resort to ordering their socks and warm clothes from a Sears Roebuck catalog.

In an effort to slow the loss of valuable surgical instruments, administrators at the third Field Hospital in Saigon bought a special metal engraver to identify the equipment. Operating room nurses spent an afternoon engraving everything only to find scissors, scalpels, and steel clamps on the Saigon streets a few days later with "3rd Field Hospital" clearly engraved across them. "I can't tell you how annoyed I was," said the army lieutenant who found the stolen supplies.

At the seventy-first Evacuation Hospital in 1970, the loss of antibiotic medication was life threatening. Soldiers burned in a plane crash filled the intensive care unit of the hospital. The antibiotic cream Sulfamylon was an essential treatment to prevent infection from overwhelming and killing these disabled men. Two nurses who worked together on that unit remember the incident. "The Sulfamylon had been stolen from the supply room. We had none at all. It was on the black market," said one of them. Her friend continued, "I wanted to get a gun and kill the marketeers for having it." Without this drug, the prognoses for the soldiers was poor. A few enlisted men went into town and reappeared with the Sulfamylon. The nurses did not ask where it came from or how they got it.

Incidents like these added to the anger and isolation the military personnel felt. Black markets were not unique to the Vietnam War—civilians have always taken advantage of abundant military supplies—but in a war where it was difficult to tell civilian from terrorist, black markets amplified suspicion and mistrust between the Americans and Vietnamese. This dubious relationship compounded the detachment many military personnel felt. The Vietnamese could not be trusted. Antiwar protesters at home condemned their work. It was never easy to live, work and fight in the war zone. What kept the participants going early in the war was the sense that the goals of the war were clear and that there was public approval for their war actions at home. However, neither of these emotional supports prevailed, and morale sagged in the final years of American involvement in Vietnam.

From 1970 to the end of 1973, when the last military nurses left the war, the pace of the action slowed and the types of patients admitted for treatment changed. Nurses saw more Vietnamese patients and more non-battle injuries. As senseless as some of the war injuries may have seemed to nurses in earlier years, the self-inflicted wounds and drug overdoses seen later in the war were even more difficult to understand. The nurses wanted to work with battle trauma, not senseless wounds or injuries. A nurse who served in Vietnam during 1971 said, "I just didn't expect to see a soldier shot from playing a game of Russian roulette or injured in a racial fight in a bar." In 1970, another nurse recalled working with twenty-nine young American men injured when an enlisted man released the safety pin on a grenade and threw it into a bar filled with fellow soldiers. She never discovered whether the attack was the result of a prank gone askew or a more sinister motive.

The esprit de corps among military personnel seemed to have vanished. It was a difficult time to be a nurse in Vietnam. The Vietnamese were not the committed allies everyone wanted. The American public opposed the war. Even some members of the military did not act as dedicated fighting troops. The women wondered what had happened to the rules they had grown with—this war did not jibe with the stories they had heard from their fathers and grandfathers.

To numb their fear and loneliness, some soldiers turned to

readily available drugs.[12] To counter the growing drug use, military leaders ordered all personnel to submit to periodic drug-screening tests. Any military personnel with positive results were immediately set home. The military was not concerned with detoxification and rehabilitation. Those recovery phases could take place stateside. Men sent home for drug problems had the option of getting treatment or receiving a "general" (not honorable) discharge from the military.[13]

Initially, government officials tried to sign contracts with commercial airlines to fly drug-positive soldiers home, but these companies refused the job. The air force took over the task of handling the "Golden Flow" flights. (This name referred to the urinalysis tests that were used to reveal drug levels.) One air force nurse in the study spent six months working on these flights. She remembered it as an unhappy time.

We flew with two armed guards in case any of the men became violent. Remember, a lot of them had not been detoxified yet and you couldn't have someone go berserk [have a drug withdrawal] at thirty thousand feet. It was too dangerous. If they did any damage to the fuselage, they would jeopardize the entire planeload of people. When we [the nurses or technicians] thought someone was going to get wild we gave them Benadryl [an antihistamine drug that causes drowsiness]. There was no fooling these guys about what pills you were giving them. They'd say to me, "Oh, you just want us to go to sleep." Their language and their lack of respect was abominable.

Some of the men on board were not drug abusers. They bought the urine of guys who were on drugs just to get home.

These men seemed willing to accept the stigma of a less than honorable military discharge rather than stay in Vietnam. After six months on "Golden Flow" flights, the nurse left the work behind.

In 1972, Henry Kissinger, National Security Adviser to President Nixon, and Le Duc Tho, head of the North Vietnamese delegation, negotiated a peace agreement at talks in Paris. On January 23, 1973, the two men reached a final agreement to end the war. Two months later, in March, the last American troops left Vietnam.[14]

Military hospitals closed. Hospital ships sailed for home. Air force nurses, however, had another wartime assignment. It was "Project Homecoming," the release of American prisoners of war from Hanoi. One nurse in the study took part in this finale to the American military involvement in Vietnam. An air force captain, she had worked on medical evacuation flights for five years. "I saw the whole war," she said. "The young kids with the war wounds. The dregs with the drug addict flights, but this last assignment, this last assignment, was the trip that made all the other work worthwhile." She had come to Vietnam with more than five years of professional experience, including nursing in the Third World. Her last job before joining the air force was as a nurse on the Project Hope hospital ship in Africa. She had volunteered for Vietnam; she had felt that it would be as exotic and challenging as her last job, and that the long hours flying patients around the world would be exciting and rewarding.

On April 1, 1973 she was part of a special crew that lifted off a runway in the Philippines. As her aircraft left for Hanoi, North Vietnam, another plane stayed behind and circled in Da Nang in the South. If the enemy shot at the first plane or if there was any mechanical trouble, the back-up plane was ready to go. Fortunately, the back-up aircraft never had to leave Da Nang.

The flight to Hanoi was very emotional for this nurse and the crew. They knew they would see Americans who had been prisoners for six, seven, and eight years. "I thought they'd [the prisoners of war] be standing in Hanoi and get all excited when they saw us [the American aircraft] land. I thought they would be ready to jump onto the plane. But you know they weren't. They were very stoic. No emotion showed at all as they walked across the tarmac to the plane." Later, the released prisoners told her that they thought their situation could change at any minute. They expected to be thrown back on a bus and taken to the Hanoi Hilton [the nickname for the grim prison where U.S. prisoners were held].[15] During their internment, the men had learned never to trust their captors. "They did not believe their freedom was ever going to come," she said.

The prisoners walked on board and quietly sat down. The aircraft prepared for departure, taxied down the runway, and lifted off. "Once the plane left the ground, the aircraft wheels went up. Remember, most of the prisoners were fliers so they knew what was happening. All of a sudden, pillows went up in the air and everyone was hollering and screaming. It was emotional; it was happy. They were going home." Eleven years later, she laughed and had tears in her eyes as she remembered those first few hours of freedom for the men.

How did the men react to her, the first American woman they had seen since their internment? "Oh," she smiled, "they wanted to know what was going on [at home] and the latest of everything. They wanted cigarettes and, of course, we stowed extra things like that and ice cream for them." The fact that she was a woman mattered less than the fact that she was an American and represented freedom. The flight from Hanoi to the Philippines went quickly. "They could not sit still. They were running up and down and talking to each other. I cried. I couldn't help it."

Once the released prisoners landed in the Philippines they received medical, psychological, and dental care and a military debriefing. After a week, these men then met the nurse again for the next part of their long trip home. "We flew to Hawaii and then we flew back to Andrews or Scott or McGuire Air Force Bases in the U.S.," she continued. "This was the final stage for them because their families were waiting for them."

The reunions were the most emotional events of her career. "You would just stand in the doorway [of the aircraft] and watch them run to their families and you would cry."

9

Leaving Vietnam

During the last three months of their tours in Vietnam, the nurses sensed a change. The war for them was ending. It was time to go home, back to the "world." The change was subtle and unconscious. Feelings and thoughts the nurses had suppressed to get through the year began to surface. They started to think about themselves again. What they discovered were a variety of feelings: fatigue, vulnerability, pride, and ambivalence.

The twelve-hour days, the heat, and the suffering had taken its toll. There was a weariness that had sapped their strength and left little energy for anything besides work and sleep. This weariness also affected their ability to sustain a strong emotional defense. As one young army nurse said, "The last three months were tough. I had been bubbly, vivacious, and optimistic. I was a strong, buoyant force, but I couldn't maintain it all. I was ready to leave."

An air force nurse mentioned that during the end of her tour she tired of getting up in the middle of the night to pick up eighteen-year-old "kids" so badly wounded they would never go home. As the women's emotional defenses faltered, the sense of wasted lives and losses mounted. There always seemed to be one more double amputee or spinal cord injury waiting for them; one more child burned with napalm.

The most common way nurses handled this emotional weight was to pull away from the work. "I didn't give as much of myself those final months. I collapsed emotionally like I had no feelings or no thoughts. I never expected it to happen to me," said one nurse who had spent ten months working in an intensive care unit. Newly arrived nurses had once turned to her for lessons. An expert clinician, she had made quick clinical decisions. At the end, however, these decisions became difficult. It was as if body and mind could no longer function in peak form. She wanted to go home.

The separation the nurses felt carried over to their personal lives. Only one nurse spoke of trying to meet new people. The others preferred to remain with familiar friends. They had said good-bye to so many people. They noticed how quickly replacements forgot their predecessors. Replacements saw their year in Vietnam stretched before them, and did not want to share in others' reminiscences. As the nurses prepared to go home, they knew that they too would soon be forgotten. It was not worth the effort to join the newcomers.

Psychologists who study this process of separation refer to it as "the termination phase," defined as, "the period of time preceding the permanent separation."[1] The phrase and related concepts evolved out of research on people in individual and group psychotherapy. At some point in treatment, people need to end their relationships with their therapists. It becomes necessary for them to move on with their lives. Clinicians now apply this concept to many different groups—students getting ready for graduation, people preparing for retirement, families relocating to another town. It is a normal process with predictable reactions. People can feel depressed, guilty, angry, or sad as they begin to move away from the familiar to the unknown.[2] Any time groups form and a member leaves, "termination" will occur.

Why did the nurses show a disinterest and withdrawal during the last three months of their tours? Were they simply "terminating" their involvement in the war? Was twelve months a natural limit for wartime nursing? How would they have reacted if the standard tour had been twenty-four months? Did they unconsciously prepare for just twelve months in the war?

Three nurses volunteered to remain in Vietnam an extra month to facilitate their military discharges. These women were allowed to leave the military earlier after they lengthened their tour. There was, however, a price to pay for their month-long extension. Each women said it had been a mistake. "Staying," said one of them, "was the worst thing I could have done. Life was hell. I felt overdue and that I was taking a chance. I should have left when the time was good." It was as if the women instinctively developed just enough emotional stamina for twelve months.

Their emotional and physical weariness may have been responsible for another feeling that began to surface in those final months. The women began to feel threatened by the war and anxious for their lives. Combat soldiers had a phrase to describe the vulnerability nurses felt: "short-timer syndrome." As a soldier neared his time to go home, he suddenly became fearful for his life and became cautious and tentative.[3] The women unknowingly shared this outlook.

Nurses who worked during enemy attacks on their compounds never gave much thought to their personal safety. But this coping strategy became ineffective as time passed. As army nurse who worked at both the twenty-fourth and the twenty-ninth evacuation hospitals in the southern part of South Vietnam described her "short-timer syndrome." She was in Vietnam from April 1968 to April 1969, during some of the fiercest battles of the war. It was in the last month of her tour that her composure left her. "The air base was attacked and all I could think about was that I was going to die before I got home. All of the attacks during the other months never bothered me but the closer I got to [going] home the more afraid I became." She was unable to sleep at night because she feared a rocket attack. She put in a request to work on the night shift. Sleep came easier during the day, when there was less chance of attack.

When the pace of the war slowed two years later, another nurse, who was stationed at a different evacuation hospital, still felt vulnerable at the end of her tour. She stopped her visits to the local orphanage. For many months before she had enjoyed the weekly trips to see the children. Now, at the end of her tour, she began to worry about being hurt by snipers or terrorists from the village. Everything seemed more menacing and more insecure. She preferred staying on the fortified military base.

Friends of these two nurses shrugged off their behavior with the phrase, "Most people get crazy when they get short."

There were times when a nurse's fear became so great that her judgment and clinical skills were affected. In one instance, a nurse lost her ability to function in a receiving ward. "It was February [during the Tet Offensive of 1968] and we were told a North Vietnamese regiment was coming towards our area. There was even small arms fire from the enemy in our compound. I slept in the bunker night after night. Actually, I didn't sleep at all." Without sleep, she lost the "edge" and her endurance. The chief nurse of the hospital transferred her to a more secure military area to await her flight home.

Home seemed so close now that the nurses could no longer deny the dangers around them. They became nervous and in doing so regained the humanity, and the vulnerability they could not afford to have in a war. It was the first step back to peacetime life.

During this final period in Vietnam, they began to receive professional respect and admiration from others. "I was a veteran. My boots and my fatigues were worn. I was teaching the newcomers. I had already been through so many experiences that nothing could come my way that I didn't know how to do." Replacements tapped this knowledge. They knew the veterans would give them the kind of knowledge no training instructor back in the states had.

Veterans taught the newcomers special clinical skills: the quickest way to insert a large needle into a man's extremities to administer intravenous fluids, or the fastest way to remove blood-soaked clothing to examine wounds, or how to make rapid, accurate triage decisions in mass casualty situations.

The new nurses in their bright green fatigues and flight suits or pressed white uniforms watched while their experienced colleagues worked through rocket attacks or storms at sea or air turbulence. They saw the veterans talk firmly to arrogant enlisted men and softly to men in pain. Finally, they listened to the personal information they would need to survive the off-duty hours. It was important to know which men to avoid dating, how to order from the Sears Roebuck catalog, the location of a well-stocked PX store, and which officers' club had the best drinks and food.

In a few months the replacements would acquire the savvy and confidence they saw in their predecessors. Soon they would be admired by another group of nurses in newly issued fatigues, thereby demonstrating the continuum of wartime nursing.[4]

The veterans enjoyed orienting the novices to the war. The sight of newcomers meant that their own time in Vietnam was limited; it assured a changing of the guard. The end was actually in sight. The veterans could feel a sense of accomplishment. They knew they had overcome any professional insecurity; they now possessed a self-confidence that comes from hard work under intense conditions; they had passed a most difficult test. And the replacements' respect verified the nurses' achievements. Here was a reward for a job well done.

Most of the nurses in the study, forty-four of the fifty women, received special citations or medals for their work. All Americans who served in the military in Vietnam between July 3, 1965 and March 28, 1973 earned two awards: the Republic of Vietnam Campaign Ribbon and the Vietnam Service Medal.[5]

Unit citations were awarded to a group of people rather than to individuals. The army nurse who set up and worked at the prisoner-of-war hospital spoke of her unit citation as one of her cherished possessions.

Each military service conferred special medals. Many army nurses received the Bronze Star. The army also gave out Commendation medals to individual nurses for special actions such as the resuscitation of a patient. Navy nurses earned Navy Achievement and Navy Commendation medals for their work. Air force nurses received Air medals for flying in a combat zone and for certain numbers of in-flight hours. One army nurse received a Purple Heart after a patient broke her jaw.

American soldiers also expressed their gratitude to the

nurses by awarding them honorary membership in their units. One nurse remembers that she was made an honorary member of the army's 101st Airborne Division.

Foreign government officials honored two nurses for their work with other nationals. One air force nurse received the Philippines Cross. An Army nurse acquired a special commendation from the Republic of Korea in appreciation for her work.

Six nurses did not get any special medals or commendations. They resented the indifference toward their efforts. Because of transfers between hospitals and commands or aloof superiors, these nurses did not receive the letters of support required for awards.

Most of the nurses are proud of the reminders of their time in Vietnam. They wear their medals on their military uniforms, display them in frames on their den walls, or keep them carefully wrapped in velvet in their jewelry boxes.

Yet one nurse, who became an ardent pacifist after the war, was embarrassed about her medals. She said that medals or any other award given for participation in war were merely tokens from an immoral time. Her feelings about medals grew out of her belief that if the military did not reward wartime work perhaps more people would be less enthusiastic about volunteering for war and risking their lives.

Nine women felt they did not deserve their medals. They said they were just doing their job in Vietnam. "I thought medals were for heroism and outstanding service. I didn't feel I did anything exceptional. I just went to work," said one nurse, referring to her Bronze Star. Another said, "We [the nurses] knew what we did. How could you justify getting a medal when the guys in the field didn't get one?" This woman and others believed in the myth that only men in combat experienced war and only those men deserved medals. They saw no valor in nursing the wounded and consoling the dying, no courage or selflessness in their work. Some of the nurses who felt undeserving of their medals faced a conflict at home. Why, then, they asked themselves, were they so unsettled by a war and a nursing experience they believed to be routine?

The nurse who received a Purple Heart illustrated how the women tended to underrate their war work. "I tried to refuse my

Purple Heart because I felt I had caused it through my own stupidity. They [the military leaders] threatened to mail it to my family. I didn't want my parents to know that I had been in danger and that I had been hurt. Instead I just got it [the medal] without a ceremony.''

Another nurse, who served between 1970 and 1971, remembered showing her medal to a soldier. Her patients included some of the last American casualties in the war. "I received a Bronze Star for my work and I showed it to an infantryman when I got home. He looked at it and began to lecture me. I got a big long story about why they gave out medals to people who were not in combat. I put it away and never looked at it again. I decided I didn't deserve it."

This nurse learned a bitter lesson about Vietnam. In the 1970s, anger toward the war and its aftermath was so great that even veterans could not recognize each other. Faced with so much criticism for their participation in an unpopular war, veterans could not reach out to one another.

At the end of their tours, the nurses became aware of their curious ambivalence toward leaving—curious because they did not expect to feel it. They thought going home would be simple. It was the day they had looked forward to for months. They imagined themselves packing up their belongings, going to their farewell parties, getting on flights home. They wanted to drive cars, go shopping, take baths, wear clothes that were not green and shoes that were not combat boots.

Many nurses drew "short-timers' calendars." These calenders, marking the last three months of their tours, often took the shape of cartoon characters. Snoopy was a favorite. At the end of each day, the short-timers colored in another small square until that last day when Snoopy finally took full shape.

Meanwhile, they thought about the friends they were leaving behind. How would these friends handle the enemy attacks and the mass casualties with only newcomers to assist them? How could they leave their patients in the hands of inexperienced nurses? The veterans felt sadness and guilt at leaving. There would be no more parties and quiet talks with friends. Their group would scatter. Reunions back home were unlikely. There would be none of the satisfaction that comes from easing pain or saving a life. No exhilarating battles to watch, no enemy attacks to survive. In a way, they would miss it. A navy nurse summed up the feelings of others when she said, "This was a time in my life that would not come again."

Their flights home were memorable, profoundly different from their flights into the war. Exuberant troops filled the airline terminals. People waited to board their "Freedom Birds," as these flights were called. Once the plane lifted off the ground, people screamed and yelled that it was over. Everyone was grateful to be alive and going home. Some nurses felt sadness as they thought about those people they knew who would never see home again.

Two nurses had unusual flights home. One of them, a navy nurse, remembered walking into a huge airline terminal in Da Nang with another woman. They were supposed to take a commercial airline home but they found out that a medical evacuation plane was leaving almost immediately. Here was an opportunity to get home sooner. They boarded the air force plane, sat down, and saw familiar faces. Some of the men lying on stretchers were their patients from the hospital ship. They all looked at each other with surprise. The nurse felt an unexpected sense of satisfaction. Here were the results of her work, the grateful faces of the men she helped save.

Another nurse also took a military flight in an effort to get home quickly. This flight was to San Francisco. It would be easy to make connections to her home town. The army nurse went on board the huge aircraft and noticed only nine other passengers. Then she turned and saw caskets in the rest of the plane. It was December 1968; that year 14,521 Americans died in Vietnam.[6]

The first glimpse of the Cascade Mountains in Washington State or the Golden Gate Bridge in San Francisco made most nurses, and the men on their flights, cry. Although some nurses had never seen the West Coast, on that day and on that flight they felt anywhere in the United States was familiar. It was real. They were home.

10

Homecoming

In Washington State or California, the nurses wearily walked down the exits and headed for the customs offices located at the military air terminals. Once they completed customs inspections, they found taxis to civilian airports. It was all routine. There were no signs, no one to say "Welcome home."

The taxi rides gave the nurses an opportunity to look at their homeland. Cars drove at fast speeds. There was no concertina wire. There were doors and pay telephones everywhere. "I went into the airport coffee shop for awhile," said one nurse. "I was amazed at the color and all the people coming and going. Baloney sandwiches and real coffee and cream! I didn't even have to sit in the back of the restaurant facing the door." Four nurses who flew home in their combat fatigues went into the first bathroom they could find and changed into civilian dresses. They threw their fatigues and combat boots into trash cans.

As children the nurses had listened to the war stories of their fathers and grandfathers. They heard about ticker-tape parades down Fifth Avenue in New York City and cheering dockside crowds in Boston and San Francisco. Embraces and tears and hugs greeted the "doughboys" and the "Yanks." As young girls, they had watched their relatives march with the local American

Legion or Veterans of Foreign War units every Fourth of July. Neighbors had waved small flags and shouted as the men went past. War veterans were American heroes.

But it was easy to dismiss the veterans who returned from Vietnam. There were no huge troop ships or airlifts. American military personnel traveled from Saigon or Da Nang alone or in small groups. They flew from the West Coast to their home towns on commercial airlines with civilians on business trips or families on vacations. On the whole, most people ignored them. Homecomings were quiet, sometimes hostile.

In the airports, nurses saw long haired hippies wearing "love beads" around their necks and old army fatigue jackets. The women felt a twinge of anger as they thought of cutting the same type of jacket off men wounded in battles. These people, the nurses thought, seemed to be mocking the sacrifice of the wounded and dead.

In the San Francisco airport, so near the college campuses where the antiwar movement blossomed, veterans and protesters mingled.[1] The two groups usually avoided contact. A fragile truce existed. Military people wanted to get home and protesters wanted their messages heard. There were times, however, when tempers flared. One nurse remembered a near fistfight between her husband, who was just off the plane from Saigon, and a group of hippies. A navy nurse saw people carrying placards with the antiwar slogan, "Hell no, we won't go." "If one of those people had come up and talked to me," she said, "I would have strangled them."

Although protesters directed their anger toward men in uniform, the nurses were not immune to harassment. Ten women in the study told stories of hostile encounters in California airports. One incident involved a navy nurse on her way home to Pennsylvania. She was alone and clearly identifiable in her blue uniform. "The whole time [in the airport] I was followed by a group of hippies who did nothing but badger me with questions. They said, 'Where have you been?,' 'What are those ribbons for?,' 'Who do you think you are?' I know I should have stood up to them but it was such a shock for me. I was so happy to be home. It was a hard way to come back."

When another navy nurse got off a plane in Los Angeles, she was knocked down by four people who called her a "fascist pig." They knocked off her glasses and quickly fled. It happened so fast, she never saw the people who hit her—or the people on the other side of the political fence who helped her up and brushed off her uniform.

She, and most other nurses, quickly learned to conceal their military affiliation. Every time they wore their uniforms off military bases, there was a chance civilians would mistreat them. For example, another woman remembered getting out of her car at home to change a flat tire. She was in her military uniform: hat, fitted jacket, skirt, stockings, and high-heeled shoes. She knew it would be difficult to use a car jack and to turn wheel bolts in her outfit so she gratefully watched a stranger slow down his car and approach her. He seemed to recognize her military uniform, because he looked at her closely and drove off without offering assistance. She removed her jacket and did the job herself.

A 1985 study by army researchers confirmed the fact that, as the war intensified, less than half (42 percent) of their sample of 361 nurses wanted other people to know they were in the army.[2] In the late sixties and seventies, a uniform was a lightning rod.

Conflicting reactions and treatment of the nurses continued on their journeys across America. The nurses also told stories about civilians showing kindness and appreciation. For example, a sympathetic flight attendant gave one nurse a free first-class airline ticket.

One army nurse, on a cross-country flight from California to New York, noticed a man in the seat next to her staring at her military uniform and her new medals, then turning away. He never said a single word to her during the six-hour flight.

As a matter of historic perspective, Vietnam veterans were not the only group of veterans who were treated as pariahs after a war. In the summer of 1932, fourteen thousand World War I veterans marched on Washington, D.C. It was the time of the Great Depression and these men were out of work. They wanted Congress to pass a bill that would pay them their bonus for wartime service. The bonus was not due to be paid until 1945. When Congress refused to act on their request, about half of the marchers went home. The other half of the war veterans were driven out of a park by the U.S. Army, men in armored tanks.[3]

After a short time at home, the nurses felt exhausted and bewildered. One army nurse remembered an incident that occurred in the New York City subway.

I had lugged my duffel bag down an escalator and over to a booth to buy a token for my ride home to Long Island. This Spanish guy [the attendant in the booth] says, "Are you in the army? Where were you?" I was very defensive. I told him that I just gotten back from Vietnam. And he said, "You were in Vietnam?" His voice was incredulous. I thought "Uh-oh, here it comes." He said "Wow," and he left his token booth. He walked up to me and said, "Let me shake your hand. I am so proud of you. My brother was there and he was wounded. Thank you for being there. Now you"—and he really emphasized that word—"get to ride the subway free today!" With that, he opened the swinging door with a flourish and let me go by.

"He was," she finished, "the only person to ever say thank-you to me in all those years."

Twenty-four hours earlier, this nurse and others had been in Vietnam with friends and patients. Unlike their predecessors from other wars, who had had weeks to conform to peacetime routine aboard ships or as they waited at embarkation points, Vietnam veterans quickly had to adjust from the jungle and the war to the American landscape. Such a rapid change of environment was jarring. The American political climate only compounded their adjustment.

As the war years continued, many military nurses adopted an alternative route home. Sixteen of the nurses in the study postponed their homecomings. They took short vacations in the Philippines or in Japan or in Hawaii. Others visited friends from Vietnam and brothers and sisters. One nurse spent two days at Disneyland—a perfect spot to escape from reality.

No one wrote of this practice in a military manual or formally suggested it during meetings. Rather, these nurses instinctively knew that they needed time to decompress before picking up their lives again. The women felt tired and needed to rest.

Their homecomings were sometimes more traumatic than their arrival at war. On the flight overseas, nurses knew they would be in a different world—a jungle, and a war zone. Going home, the women thought they were returning to the familiar. They were not. After their long journeys and their unsettling encounters, some nurses looked backed longingly to Vietnam. At least in Vietnam, they knew their place. They felt appreciated and wanted. The world made no sense anymore. No longer did the future seem so harmless. They were strangers in their homeland.

Some women felt out of step. Nurses who left the country in 1967 and 1968 for Vietnam returned home to hippies, Flower Power, Martin Luther King's and Robert Kennedy's assassinations, and turmoil on college campuses. An older women who was in her forties when she returned from Vietnam was so horrified at the antiwar slogans she saw during protest demonstrations that she chose to sleep through most of her thirty-day leave.

Many civilians seemed to be enjoying themselves. People went about their daily lives as if nothing was happening in Vietnam. The women, however, remembered their friends and the servicemen. They knew the suffering continued.

A younger nurse unexpectedly remembered the war during her first shopping trip to a mall in Connecticut. She had gone out with her sisters to buy some civilian clothes. She described the scene: "It [the mall] was so strange. The colors. Everybody seemed to be having such fun. I kept thinking about all those people I left in 'Nam. I started crying at the underwear counter."

Another nurse found herself unable to leave her house for the first two weeks she was home. "I tried to go out but I started to get very anxious. There were so many people. It was all so crazy. I just wanted to leave," she said.

Their family reunions, of course, were dramatic. "My father broke through the lines and ran to meet me at the bottom of the aircraft steps. He gave me a hug and a big twirl." The rest of her family stood crying by the airline gate. Another father, still on active duty in the military, met his daughter at the plane and saluted her. The rest of the country may have been indifferent or angry, but their families were thankful to have them back.

Their home towns soothed them with trees in full bloom and green lawns, or snow and frozen lakes. Fathers painted "Welcome Home" signs and hung them from garage doors. Mothers spent time cooking their daughters' favorite dishes. High-school and college friends stopped by with invitations to parties.

Something, however, was wrong. After the hugs and the celebratory meals, the women noticed no one wanted to hear about the war. They sensed that their parents were content to see their daughters standing in the kitchen and laughing, but war talk was another matter. It seemed as though no one wanted to upset them or be upset by their stories.

Some families carried this thinking to the extreme. For two nurses, there were no homecoming festivities. These women came home and unpacked and loudly heard the unspoken message: The war was over and it was to be forgotten. The silence seemed to diminish the importance of their war work; how much significance could it have if no one expressed any interest? Most people had different reasons for not wanting to talk about the war and encounter its veterans.

The nurses suspect a reason for their parents' silence was guilt. Perhaps after hearing one story about a dying patient or about an enemy attack, these mothers and fathers blamed themselves for exposing their daughters to such sadness and danger. Why did they let their girls volunteer for the war? Should they have been more forceful in their objections? "I sensed," said one nurse who went home to Ohio, "that my parents felt they should have prevented it [the war] somehow."

Mothers in particular seemed to want to evade the subject of war, even though, since they read news magazines and watched nightly television news, they likely knew what their children had experienced. These women preferred to talk about neighbors or wedding engagements or recent divorces. The common ground they shared with their daughters was social conversation. One nurse began to understand her mother's reaction. She said, "There was no way I could make [her] understand. I knew things she would never know. It was . . . well, very hard to talk about. Not that my memories [from Vietnam] were so horrid but it was just a sense that she wouldn't understand."

Fathers, especially those men who were also veterans, remained silent because they knew about war and how it changed people. It might have been difficult for them to think of their children, their little girls, as sullen or angry or enervated adults.

One nurse, however, broke through her father's silence. Her father, a wounded World War II marine, had dodged her war talk and it frustrated her. She tried many different avenues. Finally, he let her talk and her tales about the twelve months she spent as an intensive care nurse in the third Surgical Hospital in the Delta region of South Vietnam came flooding out. His reaction startled her. "He got tears in his eyes and he told me, 'I signed the papers so that [the war] could happen to you. I came home and I was a hero and you [Vietnam veterans] came home and you were dirt. You were my baby and I didn't want you to be hurt. . . . You were hurt and I'm sorry.' " He was able to express the guilt so many fathers, and mothers, preferred to bury.

After this encounter, the wounded ex-marine veteran of World War II became the main source of emotional support for his daughter. She relaxed and talked to him. It helped her put the Vietnam War in perspective. Six other fathers, all World War II veterans, eventually became their daughters' confidants. These talks became an opportunity to bring the men and their daughters closer together.

At night, when everyone else in the house was asleep, the fathers and daughters sat around the kitchen table and talked about "their wars," the fathers talked of the difficulties of fighting in the jungle, the daughters talked of the pathos of watching men die. They both laughed at the humor of war. They understood each other and the experience.

Another group of men, the grandfathers who served in World War I, also came to ally themselves with the nurses. One grandfather was so proud of his granddaughter's service in Vietnam that he asked for a family portrait when she returned. He put on his World War I "doughboy" uniform. She put on her army greens. Veterans from two different generations, they stood arm-in-arm before the camera.

Another grandfather spoke about his pride and gratitude. His granddaughter explained:

The only person who shared anything with me was my grandfather. He had never talked about his war. He was such a stoic German. When I came back from Vietnam, this old man comes up to me and says, "Well, now I think you've grown up," and he brought out this picture album I

had never seen before. There were pictures of a ticker-tape parade in
New York. He said, "I'm sorry it couldn't be like that for you because I
don't think the boys in Vietnam did any less than we did in World War
I." It was a grand thing for him to say.

The veteran died shortly afterward. The granddaughter
missed him all the more for their new-found camaraderie.

Family members often were not the only ones reluctant to
discuss the war. Friends, even close friends who once shared
adolescent secrets with the nurses, were suddenly like strangers.
"My friends had a surprise party for me [when I got home from
Vietnam] and not a single person asked me what I did or anything
about my experience. These were all my *best* friends. It was
just like it never happened." Some likely avoided the subject
of the war because they wanted to protect the nurses or not upset them when, in truth, often it was the listener who was simply
too timid to hear. Operating room anecdotes do not make
good party chitchat. They did not realize the women's need to
talk.

There were also political and moral reasons friends did not
want to hear about Vietnam. Some people felt that by participating in the war, the nurses showed support for a corrupt government. The nurses sensed that to bring up the subject of war might
be to instigate a heated political debate. Their friends, particularly men, often felt guilty that the nurses, women, answered the
government's summons while they, men, stayed home to work or
to go to school. Talking about Vietnam made them feel inferior,
even cowardly. Facing this silence made one nurse, an army
veteran who returned home to northern New York state, angry.
"Everything that I didn't want to come back to happened . . . I
wanted to grab people and say, 'Don't you care? Your own
people are being mutilated and tortured and killed and you don't
even care.' I was angry at my friends. I couldn't identify with
them. I was very disappointed and I still feel that way to some
extent."

The reaction of their friends made the nurses aware of a
change in their lives: a space would always exist between those
who had been to war and those who had stayed home. One army

nurse said, "I went to see my friends and they didn't want to hear about Vietnam. I couldn't relate to them. I thought people had to know what was going on over there but people didn't want to hear it. I started to feel really alienated."

The sense of estrangement was not unique to Vietnam veterans. People who had returned from other wars had met the same treatment. Theresa Archard, a captain in the army nurse corps during World War II, wrote in 1945:

Now that I was back in the States again, my reaction to the surroundings and people was perhaps typical of those who return from combat areas—so many people insensitive to the reality of a world at war and its tragedies beyond number, concerned only with the way it might be inconveniencing them. I was heartsick when I thought of the boys in the tent hospitals. . . . Yet people at home complained of a shortage of luxuries.[4]

The average citizen had never suffered from acute shortages or feared for his or her life and home. It was difficult for people at home to be committed to a war far away. Veterans often misinterpreted this indifference as a sign of disloyalty to those who gave so much.

After suffering disaffection, only five of the fifty nurses continued to talk about Vietnam. The rest chose to keep their feelings and experiences hidden. One nurse deliberately did not answer her telephone the first year she was home from Vietnam. She simply did not want to answer thoughtless questions or hear antiwar comments.

Of course, there was always an audience for the funny stories and the exotic travel tales, but most nurses chose to conceal the core, the real substance of the Vietnam experience. Why should they share such an intense and special experience with uncaring individuals? "People would say to me, 'What was it like in Vietnam?' and then turn away before I could say anything," said a former navy nurse. "The war meant something to me. It had a great impact on me and I just did not want to share it [the war] with people who didn't want to know." Many other women agreed with her. "People's disinterest hurt me. I'd rather they didn't know because it was too personal,'' said another nurse who remained in the military after the war.

The American public had become saturated with the subject of Vietam.[5] On nightly television, they had seen firefights and wounded men on ponchos being dragged to helicopters. Television anchormen reported the weekly casualty figures from Vietnam with the same tone of voice they reported stock market figures. Why would anyone want to hear more stories about the war?

The nurses resented the indifference to their own experiences; they also found the public apathy disturbing. "It was the first television war, and I guess people got fed up with it. I became very concerned with an American public who can watch TV and say, 'Oh, my, eight people got killed in Vietnam today. What else is on TV?' What happened to feeling and caring for each other?'' said one woman who stopped trying to talk about the war.

Some nurses thought that people who have never been to war would never fully understand the experience, that war was an ordeal outside any normal human event, one that cannot be captured in a brief explanation. As one woman said, "When people said, 'What was it like?' What a silly open-ended question! I couldn't really answer them.''

The result of all this silence on the part of many women was the postponement of any personal analysis of the Vietnam war. They never reconciled their memories of Vietnam with their lives after the war. The two worlds remained separate. Some nurses lived, even flourished, in one world while they kept the other buried. A basic conflict emerged from these segmented lives. The nurses were proud of their time at the war, but were unable to acknowledge it—to publicly declare it. No one wanted to hear.

Many of the nurses in this study remained isolated. One woman who stayed in the military said she spent four years in the same office with another nurse who served in Vietnam—they worked together every day—but they never once talked about the war.

In 1984, at the time of these interviews, the silence was about to break. Nurses were planning reunions with their comrades. Someone was writing an annual newsletter with the news and addresses of all the hospital personnel who served at the twelfth

Evacuation Hospital in Cu Chi. Even the public had begun to listen. "Some of the younger nurses I work with now ask me questions [about Vietnam]. They seem genuinely interested," said one navy nurse who now frequently discusses her work at NSA Da Nang in 1969.

Slowly, the veterans had begun to shed their mistrust.

11
The Years Since the War

More than half of the women interviewed for this study chose to remain in the military. This world was a familiar one. Military life offered professional advancement and a solid career. Twelve women stayed on active duty. Fifteen others opted for reserve duty, which required one weekend a month and two weeks a year of active duty. They all received an unexpected benefit from their decision to accept another commission: the military provided a sense of camaraderie the civilian world did not.

Friendships among people in the postwar service never reached the intensity they had in Vietnam, but the Vietnam veterans did share an unspoken bond and acceptance. Veterans wore the two easily recognizable Vietnam service ribbons on their uniforms every day. As one nurse who chose to stay in the Navy Nurse Corps said, "The ribbons always caught your eye and immediately both of you knew you shared a part of each other's past without ever knowing anything else."

This recognition did not mean that veterans would sit down and swap war stories. More likely, they would just nod or ask each other what year and where they were stationed in Vietnam before moving on. Still, these brief contacts helped the nurses feel less isolated. "It's not that we talked about Vietnam," said one. "We didn't have to talk about it. There was a sense that we knew where we all had been."

In contrast, the women who left the military often found themselves the only Vietnam veteran in their group of friends or in their workplace or in their neighborhood.

Twenty-three nurses returned to civilian life. Four of the women left the military immediately after Vietnam. These four look back with regret at the sudden transition. In their haste to muster out of the service, they had not considered the consequences of quickly severing strong ties. One nurse who resigned her officer's commission in San Francisco less than a week after coming home said, "It's not something I would recommend for anybody in the future. We were so surrounded by Vietnam and the camaraderie. It was like getting a divorce." In hindsight, she added, she wished she had spent another two-year tour in the military before becoming a civilian.

The other nineteen nurses spent short periods of time—from two to nine months—completing their military service. On their last day in service the women went through the standard procedure for military discharge: they signed a form stating they did not wish to remain on active duty; they returned all military equipment; they read and signed a paper acknowledging that they understood the GI Bill of Rights; and, finally, they received their last paycheck. Once home, they stored their military uniforms in the attic, next to their prom dresses and student nurse uniforms.

Working in stateside military hospitals helped nurses ease into peacetime life. Most of their patients there were recuperating from wounds received in Vietnam. Yet, although the wards were filled with familiar sights and sounds, the relationship between the nurses and their patients had changed. Now, nurses and patients were both veterans. They talked about their futures and kept the camaraderie of the war alive.

Three nurses met patients they had cared for in Vietnam. These meetings completed a cycle; they were able to see the results of their nursing care. A young navy nurse remembered her first stateside assignment in the open-heart unit at Bethesda Naval Hospital. One day, as she sat at the nurses' desk writing notes on her patients, she looked down and saw a pair of shiny black shoes. "It's obviously a marine," she thought. She looked up at him and saw a smiling young man in uniform. She did not recognize his face, yet clearly he knew her and wanted to talk. "You know," he began, "I've been waiting for you to come back. I want to thank you for taking care of me." She could not guess how he had found her, but to this nurse his appreciation represented that of all the patients she had cared for in Vietnam.

Other nurses ended up working with patients undergoing reconstructive surgery for bones shattered in Vietnam. They watched men learn to walk again and hoped their other former patients were also recuperating somewhere with newly rebuilt jaws and hands and knees.

On two occasions nurses discovered patients they had thought were dead. "This guy lost his eyes, his legs, his right arm and he had chest and belly wounds. Nobody expected him to live. He didn't have a prayer. He was med-evaced [transferred] off the ship. I got to the Philadelphia Naval Hospital and here was this same guy walking on his stumps. I can remember my eyes filling up that day. He remembered my voice."

Returning to work at either military or civilian hospitals after the war required an adjustment back to the subservient roles nurses performed in the United States. In their rush to get back home, the nurses did not stop to consider the disparity between nursing practice in war and peace. At that time, the profession was just beginning to achieve autonomy, but for the most part, physicians and hospital administrators dictated how nurses practiced their work.[1] This structured environment was very different from Vietnam.

In war their professional skills gave them a certain autonomy. The nurse's role was clear and basic—to provide physical and emotional care to patients. A nurse's ability to assess a change in neurological status often saved a life, or a nurse's ability to comfort a newly disabled young soldier provided the basis for the man's psychological rehabilitation.

But in civilian hospitals, they could not function professionally the way they had done in the war. Eight nurses spoke about the difficult time they had dealing with the bureaucratic constraints stateside. In Vietnam, they said, a nurse's skill was appreciated. There was a mutual professional regard between physician and nurse. It was difficult for them to surrender their autonomy and accept the male dominated medical system of the civilian world. In the United States, nurses saw themselves slip into the traditional role of a handmaiden. One nurse, who had helped assess and perform initial treatment on wounded soldiers in an evacuation hospital in South Vietnam, returned to a North Carolina hospital. She related, "I questioned a doctor and got reprimanded. It was like a slap in the face, and I saw all my powers taken away from me." In the end, she decided to retire from nursing and now spends her time raising a family in the suburbs of New York City.

Seven women who shared her views have stayed in the profession, but they are now in supervisory or independent-practitioner positions where they are no longer subjected to the direct authority of physicians. These women felt that, after Vietnam, they were never again able to practice with the same level of responsibility, authority, or skill. In a broader sense, they question the general role and practice of nurses in America. One nurse, who now is a medical-surgical supervisor in a hospital, summed up the feelings of the other nurses: "If only nursing could be the way it was practiced in Vietnam when you were appreciated for all your skills. I like nursing, but I don't like the way it is practiced today."

Not all the nurses in this study shared this disillusionment. The other forty-two nurses said their feelings about nursing practice were unaffected by the war. The reactions of these women were somewhat puzzling, given the dramatic changes in the way they were allowed to practice.

Authors Margaret R. Higonnet and Patrice L. R. Higonnet provide some explanation for the nurses' impassiveness. In peacetime, they argue, each gender typically performs specific roles that are determined by society and its cultural norms. In wartime, however, women take on roles previously reserved for men. The nurses in Vietnam, for example, found themselves in positions of authority usually assumed by male physicians. In postwar life, the women reverted to the status quo and submitted to the authority of men.[2] The reversion of these nurses to their traditional roles was not a conscious decision; they simply did what was expected of them according to cultural norms that for them had not been called into question.

No matter how each nurse felt about the practice of nursing at home, all had professional decisions to make: should they stay in nursing or change professional careers? Three women chose to leave nursing and pursue other work. They said their year in Vietnam did not affect their choices. One woman had never planned a career in nursing and the other two simply found better career opportunities in other fields. All three women work in business ventures: one on Wall Street, one with a health care corporation, and one as a founder of an employee consulting firm. "I'm not the same person who decided to go into nursing. I have different needs now that my current job fulfills," noted one of the former nurses.

A second decision the nurses faced was, if they remained in nursing, where were they going to work? Would they stay in the specialty areas in which they had become so expert in Vietnam? Or would they move to a different area of nursing?

Their experience in the war directly affected the way forty-three of the nurses in this study approached their choice of clinical work. These women changed their area of nursing for one or a combination of four reasons: they no longer wanted to get involved with patients; they found it difficult to be sympathetic to civilian patients after working with war-wounded soldiers; they had seen enough suffering and death; they wanted to work with psychiatric rather than physical ailments.

Some changed because they could no longer deal with patients and their problems. It was as if the intensity of wartime nursing had used up their emotional resources—a problem described some years after the war as "burnout."

A nurse with many years of experience before the war spent twelve months in Vietnam as an operating-room—recovery-room nurse working with wounded marines. She recalls her return to work after the war. "I always loved nursing, but I had a hard time dealing with patients when I came back. Maybe I could do it now, but I couldn't for a long time." Memories of working with the wounded overwhelmed her ability to perform. After the war, she chose to work as a nursing administrator for a major health concern in the United States, where she has been highly successful.

Others changed their areas of specialty because they no longer looked on human suffering in the same way. After spending a year working with grievous war injuries, some nurses found it difficult to be sympathetic to people recovering from routine surgeries. One nurse remembers, "I tried to go back to intensive care but I couldn't. I found myself not being able to respond to people recuperating from gallbladder surgery. I felt they had no right to complain about pain. On some level I knew I was wrong but I couldn't help it." This woman left critical care nursing and has worked in various staff and administrative medical-surgical positions since the war.

Another nurse, who stayed in the military, recalled her return to work. "When I first came home I'd see a trauma patient and think 'That's not bad, they'll get well.' I almost developed a casualness about how people can be badly injured and survive. I also had no patience with whiny patients. I remember thinking, 'I've had people shot up from head to toe and they don't complain an iota. You've got a sliver and you're yelling up a storm.' I left ICU and went into geriatrics."

This group of nurses had become accustomed to a different standard of suffering. In the years since the war, their perspective has softened and some have come to understand their initial reactions to stateside patients. Still, their initial reactions changed the course of their professional careers.

Others changed their clinical focus because, as one nurse who had worked in a receiving (emergency room) in Vietnam put it, "I had had enough." They wanted to function in a more health-oriented nursing specialty. A nurse who worked in intensive care in Vietnam and who is now an administrator in a geriatric facility said, "At first [after the war], I worked in maternity to get far away from dying people. I wanted to see life starting out. Now I work in geriatrics because I can deal with death at the end of life. All those twenty-year olds—death in geriatrics seems easier, reasonable, and more acceptable to me."

Another woman, who left critical care and became a nurse-practitioner in a university student health center as a direct result of the war, said, "Today I'm working with the same age group as my patients in Vietnam. But unlike the war, I can keep this group of young people alive and healthy."

Other nurses who felt the same way are working in birth control clinics, out-patient clinics, and rehabilitation centers—places where they are unlikely to see people die.

Finally, four nurses changed their professional focus because of an interest they developed during the war. These women noticed the emotional as well as physical reactions in their patients in Vietnam. They wanted to understand the psychological reaction to injury. One nurse who now teaches at a university said, "My entire career changed as a result of the war. Vietnam triggered an interest in me to study psychiatric reactions to events." This nurse and the others went on to graduate work in psychiatric nursing in order to obtain the skills they would need to work in this area. Two of these nurses returned to their original group of patients. They provide counseling for male Vietnam veterans who have emotional problems.

Those nurses who did not change their area of nursing have taken advantage of their war experience. Those who were inexperienced before the war developed their skills and later felt confident with critically ill patients. A woman who works with cardiac patients said, "I never would have ventured into intensive care on my own, but the war taught me to be challenged by complex, difficult patients." One nurse who still works in an emergency room said she is respected for her ability to handle stress. "There is no injury that can come through the hospital doors that is worse than what I saw in Vietnam." Other nurses speak of the fact that their Vietnam experience exposed them to new areas of nursing they might not have seen at home in their local hospitals. These women still work as neurosurgery, orthopedic, and operating room nurses. They came to enjoy the challenges.

Some nurses who stayed in the military remained close to their war experiences in other ways. Four nurses in the study fly on air evacuation planes. They use their expertise to train other nurses in flight work. They serve as role models for a new generation of nurses.[3]

The navy nurse corps called on three veterans for assistance in designing new hospital ships. A number of nurses in the army used their experiences to train and develop plans for nurses in war situations. One women has spent the last eight years teaching nurses how to set up and use combat support or mobilization hospitals. "I try to use my nursing experience in Vietnam to plan what we have to do. It will probably still be a shock [for inexperienced nurses], but at least they will be a little prepared. I use my experience to help them deal with what they would face in war.''

Four women in the study felt their wartime experiences did not affect their career decisions. One of these women is still in the military. She views her Vietnam experience as a natural part of the progression of her military career. The other two nurses are involved in medical-surgical nursing and intensive care—personal preferences, not based on the past.

After the war, most of the nurses planned to return to school for undergraduate or advanced degrees. Eleven received bachelor's degrees in nursing; twenty obtained master's degrees in nursing; and eight nurses earned master's degrees in related fields. Their degrees in business and management helped them further careers as supervisors, educators, and directors of nursing. Four nurses in the study completed doctoral degrees—an unusually high number. In a 1986 federal report on the status of nursing, researchers noted there were 1.6 million registered nurses in the United States but only 4,108, or less than one quarter of one percent of the total nurses, held doctoral degrees.[4] The availability of military and veteran's benefits may help account for the high level of education among the veteran nurses.

In the course of returning to school, nurses, of course, confronted Vietnam. "It was difficult to go to graduate school and listen to the professor talk anti-Vietnam," said a woman who remained in the military. "I remember thinking that 'you don't know what you are talking about.'" This nurse chose to speak out against her professor. He reacted with surprise, as most people did, that women had served in Vietnam. He listened to her, but she doubted that his views changed. Colleges across the country in the late 1960s and early 1970s were filled with students who had stayed in school to avoid the draft. Only one other nurse said she answered antiwar activists. This woman told them stories of the results of the Viet Cong atrocities she had seen while serving at the eighteenth Surgical Hospital in Quang Tri. She was attempting to balance the horror stories she had heard about American soldiers and to protect their reputations—in essence, she was still trying to take care of her patients.

Some nurses were harassed on college campuses. At UCLA, students asked a nurse where her last job had been. She told them she had worked on a surgical orthopedic ward. When she mentioned where she had worked—in Nha Trang—they began to ask her one of the favorite rhetorical questions of the popular antiwar movement: how many people did you kill? The atmosphere on campus, and anywhere else where the antiwar movement was strong, set up a conflict for the nurses: they were proud of their year in the war, but able to acknowledge that fact to very few. The silence they chose to observe in dealing with friends and family extended over into their public lives.

Five nurses elected to join the antiwar movement. The anger they felt over the senseless loss of young lives drove them to march under the banner of protest. A woman who worked with wounded soldiers in an intensive care unit at an evacuation hospital came to see the war as morally wrong. Becoming involved in the antiwar movement seemed the logical outlet for her, and she joined the Vietnam Veterans Against the War (VVAW). Formed by returned male veterans, this group is best remembered for a rally held in 1971 in Washington, DC, where VVAW members threw their war medals on the steps of the U.S. Capitol to demonstrate their opposition to the war.[5]

Five nurses in the study went to rallies and joined the calls for peace and troop withdrawal. Eventually, each nurse left the VVAW or took an inactive role. The nurse who worked in the evacuation hospital and joined the VVAW to express her anger explained: "I was making a speech [at one of the VVAW rallies] and I had to stop. I mean I just stopped talking. I thought I was betraying all those men. I was betraying all the people I had taken care of." Once again, the professional fell back on her creed. In the end, the nurses remained advocates for the warriors, not for the war, but it was hard to speak against the latter without betraying the former.

All wars, even unpopular ones, focus on male soldiers while the nurses work unseen, out of view. While researching her book, *The Nun's Story,* author Kathryn Humle learned about a motto painted above the doorway of a convent hospital in Belgium for all nurses to see. The slogan captured the tradition of quiet, anonymous dedication that was expected from the profession. It read "Do good, and disappear."

Early in the 1970s, a nurse who enrolled at the University of Connecticut repeatedly met people who did not believe she was a veteran. She had left the army nurse corps and used the GI Bill to pay for her tuition and living expenses. Each semester she applied for these benefits and each semester she received the same reaction. She explained, "I would go to the veterans' affairs office and tell them I've come to apply for the GI Bill. They would ask me if this was for my husband. I'd tell them, 'No, it's for me.' The guys in the office looked surprised. 'You were in Vietnam?' I'd say, 'Yes.' Then these men would laugh and wink at me and say, 'Where were you when we were there? We didn't see anybody who looked like you!' It was always embarrassing for me." These comments played off the myth that women who volunteered for military duty, especially in a war zone, were surrounded and wooed by legions of men.[6]

Official large scale research on Vietnam veterans omitted nurses. The U.S. Senate Committee on Veterans' Affairs commissioned a study to examine the peacetime adjustments of veterans. In the sample of twelve hundred veterans, not a single women was included.[7] A 1980 Louis Harris Poll was conducted to assess public attitude toward Vietnam era veterans. Researchers interviewed twenty-four hundred Vietnam veterans or men who served in the military during the Vietnam era.[8] Not a single women was interviewed.

National veterans' organizations had relegated women to auxiliary membership. The one exception to this rule was the largest of the Vietnam veterans' organizations, the Vietnam Veterans of America (VVA), which has always included women as active members. A former army nurse who served in Vietnam, Mary Stout, is currently the president of this organization.

One nurse returned home to Pennsylvania and tried joining a traditional veterans' group. "At one time I approached a VFW [Veterans of Foreign Wars] guy and said, 'Hey, I'm a Vietnam veteran and maybe I'll come and join your group.' And he said to me, 'No, you can't. We don't let women in.' 'The hell with you,' she shot back, 'I never wanted to join it anyway.'"

Even the government agency whose mission was to assist veterans did not respond to the women. In a 1982 report to Congress, the director of a federal study on access to veterans' benefits noted that the Veterans Administration had not focused on the needs of women. The report was particularly critical of insufficient medical facilities. The director of the study cited the case of a San Francisco VA medical center as an example of bureaucratic oversight. Ten women were denied out-patient care for nonservice-connected problems at the San Francisco hospital during the first five months of 1982, whereas the medical needs of men with nonservice-connected problems were routinely met.[9]

Until the mid-1980s, the nursing profession did not acknowledge the Vietnam veterans in its ranks. Civilian nurses had the same reactions as the public: they ignored Vietnam veterans or they disapproved of their support for the war. Three nurses told about the reactions of colleagues who knew they were veterans. One veteran's nursing supervisor said she would set up a program to allow the nurse to show her slides and talk about her work in Vietnam, but the supervisor ultimately never planned the program. In another instance, younger nurses asked a veteran to tell them about the parties, rather than the work, in Vietnam. Finally, a third woman found herself labeled "supernurse": People expected her to do everything with precision and confidence. No one felt a need to help her because they thought she had done it all at war. This attitude isolated her from her peers.

In 1984, two former army nurses from Minnesota and Wisconsin proposed a monument honoring women who served in Vietnam. They founded the Vietnam Women's Memorial Project. The prototype statue, which they hope will eventually stand in Washington, D.C., is a woman dressed in combat fatigues; she has a stethoscope around her neck and bandage scissors sticking out of a pocket. This project seemed to have awakened professional interest in nurse veterans. The American Nurses Association and other professional organizations have announced support for the project. Nurses all over the country have donated money. In 1989, the two founders are still awaiting approval to erect the statue.[10]

Some nurses discovered a kind of kinship with male Vietnam veterans they met at school. Others found support in the veterans they dated or married. A few kept in touch with the people they served with in the war.

Nurses often noticed the other veterans in their classes. The men, recipients of GI Bill benefits, were slightly older than the average undergraduate and often took a more serious approach to their studies. Occasionally, a woman veteran would notice a limp or a scar. These men, like the nurses, learned to hide the fact that they had served in an unpopular war. They, too, wanted to get on with their lives.

When Vietnam veterans met in college, it was usually informal and without fanfare. One woman, an older career military nurse, found herself with other veterans on a Maryland campus. Initially, she made a connection with another student in an undergraduate course. The student was "a nice young man," and they became friends. "When he found out I was in Vietnam, we really talked. He introduced me to other veterans and sometimes we'd have a little group and sit and chat about what happened in the war." This group and others were a buffer to a sometimes hostile civilian world. Veterans understood the need for mutual support long before the Veterans Administration officially opened its Vet Centers for counseling and support.

Half of those interviewed (twenty-five nurses), married or became involved with male Vietnam veterans. There was little agreement among them about the support they received in such relationships.

Most of the women, sixteen of the twenty-five, felt their men helped them adjust. A navy nurse who married a man she met while serving on the USS *Repose* said, "It would be hard for me to marry someone who didn't understand or couldn't relate to what I'd been through." Another woman, a former army nurse who never married, recently realized that all her serious relationships, with one exception, were with Vietnam veterans. "I don't know why," she said. "I feel very comfortable with them because they understand something about me that I can't even define for myself." Perhaps it was a collective past, a common knowledge of fear, excitement, fatigue, anger, sadness, and loss.

The other nine women have not found their husbands or cohabitants supportive. One army nurse, married to a veteran for almost seventeen years, said, "He doesn't talk about Vietnam. It's hard for me because I want to tell him how I feel. But there is a wall there. We don't fight or argue about it, but our marriage contains a keep-off-the-grass-sign when it come to the war. It's strange, but we talk about the funny stuff. When it comes to the gut-wrenching stuff, he won't talk or listen.''

Another woman lived with a veteran for seven years. When she and her boyfriend got together with friends who served in Vietnam, they reduced the war to comic burlesque. ''I must have told mine [her war stories] a hundred times [over the years], but never never with feelings.''

A third nurse married a man who had served in Vietnam before her. They wrote to each other while she was overseas and married and had a child shortly after she came home. ''I love my husband very much. But I married him because I didn't want to be alone when I got home [from Vietnam]. I was terrified of being alone. A lot of guys came back and got married immediately and I was no different. I was terrified at having to go out and start a social life.'' After their marriage, something was missing. ''I never talk about it [the war] and he never talks about it. He's very threatened by my experience over there. Primarily because I was over there with all those men.''

Other men shared her husband's insecurity about women who went to war. They, too, did not want to hear the nurses' stories. One husband, described as ''a sensitive man,'' did not want to know where his wife served in Vietnam. For men who did not go to Vietnam, there was a clear reversal of roles. She was a war veteran; he was not. She had experienced the traditional male rite of passage. He had not.

Some nurses on the job found themselves under fire from men who had not served. ''The men where I work kidded me about being a colonel. I served in Vietnam and they didn't. I think they were uncomfortable,'' said one nurse, who chose to minimize the importance of her war work for the sake of on-the-job harmony. Another nurse noticed that her husband, who was never in the military, bristled when friends teased him about his wife wearing combat boots. He disliked watching her slide shows from the war. She thought her boldness, her war adventure, threatened him.

Three women in the study married men they met in Vietnam only to watch their marriages fall apart in the years after the war.

One nurse married a helicopter pilot. Another married a technician who flew air evacuation flights with her. A third nurse married a man from her social circle at the third Surgical Hospital in
Dong Tam.

One of these women talked about the dissolution of her wartime marriage.

We were married three years when we separated and five years when
we divorced. The basis of our relationship formed in another world
and it didn't convert. It's not the same. You're incredibly needy of
each other there and not so needy here. Of course, other factors
played a part. I don't know if we had met each other here if we
would have still gotten divorced but—my divorce is my casualty from
Vietnam.

These divorces, of course, only added to their sense of loss.
Some were left wondering if there was any reward or any good at
all to come out of the war.

The only sure payoff, it turned out, was in the lasting friendships that developed between some of the nurses. These relationships were their succor. The friendships that began in the hospital
wards, the receiving wards, the ship wardrooms, and the aircraft
hangers often developed into a deep affection that has survived
time and distance.

It was not an easy task to keep contacts alive at home. Those
nurses who became civilians found that personal changes and the
stigma associated with the war forced them and their friends
apart. Reunions of Vietnam veterans were not popular in the
1970s. At first, there were telephone calls, letters, and invitations
to weddings. After a few years, the contacts came only in a card
at Christmas. Sometimes the card contained news of a new child
or house or job, but often there was simply just a wistful sentence
about maybe getting together next year.

One former army nurse and her veteran husband organized a
reunion of the twelfth Evacuation Hospital five years after they
came home. More than 150 people, many with children, attended
the weekend event. This unit remained unusually cohesive. Each
year, they circulate a newsletter at Christmas with names, ad-

dresses, and news. Periodically, the nurses, doctors, hospital administrators, laboratory technicians, and corpsmen get together.

Three nurses in the study who worked and lived in Pleiku at the seventy-first Evacuation Hospital recently linked up again. They all left the army nurse corps when their tours ended and quietly moved into civilian work. They reunited through contacts made in an unofficial network of military nurses that came about in the early 1980s, when male Vietnam veterans began to receive public recognition. Lynda Van Devanter, a former army nurse who also served in Pleiku, started this informal group. She was the women veterans' coordinator for the Vietnam Veterans of America and the author of a popular book about her war experience, *Home Before Morning*.

One nurse who served at the twenty-fourth Evacuation Hospital in Long Binh in 1971 and 1972 used to scan the *Army Times* newspaper to see if anyone from her unit was planning a gathering. She believes that the bonds among her wartime friends could be reestablished. "I think that once we got over what we've been doing for the last fifteen to seventeen years, the old comfort feeling would return." She and others long for the old intimacy.

Ten nurses who stayed in the military regularly hold reunions with their friends. In the initial gatherings, everyone relived their most humorous moments. During later reunions, people talked about the more painful times. The nurses felt these gatherings were the homecomings the nation never gave them.

As the years pass, the nature of their friendships have changed. They began tending one another's children. They helped one another with schoolwork. They "networked" with each other's careers. Eventually, a few nurses moved into powerful positions. Those nurses who achieved the highest military ranks never forgot their friends from Vietnam. One woman assumed a leadership position in Washington, D.C. "I cannot be objective to the people I served with. If someone reports them, I can only think in terms of what happened [in Vietnam] and I can forgive them anything." Like military men who have developed a brotherhood and support classmates from an academy, shipmates, or aircraft crew members, women have their own club, their own allegiance.

Not every nurse yearned to keep in touch with wartime friends. One woman felt that reunions reminded people of the dead. "Some people said, 'Let's have a reunion of the people we were at Fort Bragg with.' I said no because I didn't want to go to a reunion and see all the ones who are missing. Ignorance is bliss and my life needs to go on."

12

Coming to Terms with the War: Post-Traumatic Stress Disorder

The nurses who served in Vietnam thought their work would be just another professional job—more intense and more exciting perhaps but, they reasoned, nursing was nursing. Wartime literature and movies had reinforced this belief. Books such as *G.I. Nightingale* (1945) and *A Nurse's War* (1979), the movie *So Proudly We Hail* (1943), and the 1970s television series "M*A*S*H" all showed nurses functioning and surviving in war zones. During the Vietnam War, U.S. Army General Neel reported, "The highest quality of nursing care was given despite the constant threat of attack."[1]

One exception to this notion of normalcy was Vera Brittain's account of her first years in England after World War I, *Testament of Youth*.

"Try as I would to conceal my memories, the War obstinately refused to be forgotten; and by the end of the Easter term [she was a student at

Oxford], 1920, its extraordinary aftermath had taken full possession of my warped and floundering mind . . . [t]he horrible delusion, first experienced after the flight from Girton, that my face was changing, persisted until it became a permanent fixed obsession."

I have since been told that hallucinations and dreams and insomnia are normal symptoms of over-fatigue and excessive strain, and that, had I consulted with an intelligent doctor after the War, I might have been spared the exhausting battle against nervous breakdown which I waged for 18 months. But no one, least of all myself, realized how near I drifted towards the point of craziness. I was ashamed, to the point of agony, of the sinister transformation. . . . Nothing has ever made me realize more clearly the thinness of the barrier between normality and insanity than the persistent growth like an obscene, overshadowing fungus, of these dark hallucinations throughout 1920.[2]

Psychologists today call this psychological reaction "post-traumatic stress disorder" (PTSD); it is defined as a syndrome that becomes evident in the aftermath of a traumatic event that is outside the usual range of human experience.[3]

The concept of PTSD is not new. In 1666, Samuel Pepys described the reaction he suffered after the Great Fire of London. His symptoms fall into the classic PTSD pattern; he felt numb and had nightmares for months after fires destroyed much of central London.[4] Sigmund Freud and his colleague J. Breuer thought PTSD was a "traumatic hysteria" that occurred after a psychic trauma. Freud and Breuer postulated that memories of an event normally faded in time as people vented their emotions, tempered their traumatic memory, or came to associate the event with more positive or comforting thoughts, but that if stressful memories were suppressed, hallucinations or attacks of hysteria occurred.[5]

The two world wars provided researchers and clinicians with large numbers of people who, as a result of their activities on the battlefield, were unable to function in everyday postwar life. During World War I, psychologists referred to PTSD as "shell shock";[6] in World War II, they called it "combat fatigue."[7] In 1945, Grinker and Spiegel studied army airmen and developed a list of the nineteen most common symptoms seen in men after they were removed from combat. These symptoms included restlessness, irritability, fatigue, and difficulty falling asleep. The researchers concluded that the symptoms resulted from a failure to adapt to the rigors of war.[8] The same nineteen symptoms are considered indicative of PTSD today.

A review of the literature on shell shock and combat fatigue indicated that researchers excluded from their work nurses who served in combat areas.[9] Following World War II, however, researchers began to study the phenomenon in increasingly diverse populations. They studied survivors of the Hiroshima bomb blast, survivors of the Holocaust, and victims of the Coconut Grove nightclub fire.[10] Two major conclusions emerged from this later work: first, that people other than combat soldiers suffered from debilitating psychological reactions, and second, stress reactions could appear long after an event ended. Psychologists found that symptoms from traumatic events could be delayed or could develop into chronic problems.

In 1975, Horowitz and Solomon predicted that large numbers of male Vietnam veterans would suffer from stress reactions in future years. They observed behavior at various Veterans Administration hospitals and concluded that many men had unresolved feelings about Vietnam. Returning to civilian life would cause these emotions to surface, they wrote. They referred to the veterans' reaction as "delayed stress response syndrome."[11]

Later research on male Vietnam veterans confirmed Horowitz and Solomon's prediction. Studies indicated that one-quarter to one-half of all male veterans suffered symptoms of PTSD for many years after their return home. Men who had seen a high degree of combat and men without a stable home life were at the greatest risk of developing a stress syndrome.[12]

Public awareness to the stress reactions of male Vietnam veterans began after the *New York Times* published a story about a Medal of Honor recipient who was killed in a Detroit robbery attempt three years after his return from Vietnam. The reporter noted the veteran had been treated for depression caused by "post-Vietnam adjustment problems."[13]

By the late 1970s, PTSD or delayed stress response, was a label that carried a stigma. It was associated with people who could not adjust to peacetime life, social failures, and malcontents. Men who were truly troubled by the war and carried the burden of the disorder did not realize that their fathers and grandfathers, the heroes from World Wars I and II, also had suffered.

Many veterans who needed help avoided it for fear of being labeled with a mental disorder.[14]

Official recognition of this stress reaction occurred in 1980, when the American Psychological Association included the disorder in the third version of their main diagnostic reference manual—the *Diagnostic and Statistical Manual (DSM III).*—where it gained the designation of post-traumatic stress disorder (PTSD). Three subtypes of PTSD were cited: acute PTSD, which occurs immediately after the stressful event; chronic PTSD, wherein individuals experience symptoms for six months or longer; and delayed PTSD, wherein sufferers have an onset of symptoms six months or longer after the event has ended.[15] Inclusion in the *DSM* legitimized and standardized diagnoses of emotional reaction to all types of traumas, including those experienced in the Vietnam war.

Until 1982, when Schnaier released the results of a research study examining the nurses' experience in Vietnam, knowledge about the presence of PTSD in women veterans populations was speculative. The Schnaier study, however, and another report by Paul and O'Neill, both indicated that one-quarter of their samples (made up of nurses who served in Vietnam) suffered from PTSD at the time the studies were conducted.[16]

Stretch, Vail, and Mahoney, a team of army researchers, found much lower levels of PTSD in their sample of Vietnam veteran nurses. They noted a current PTSD rate of 3.3 percent.[17] One reason for the discrepancy in those findings may be that the Schnaier and Paul studies for the most part involved nurses who left the military, while the Stretch study included only women still on active duty in the Army Nurse Corps. These two distinct groups of respondents live in very different environments. The amount of emotional support, the recognition for their war work, and personal reasons for taking part in these research studies probably varied greatly between members of the military and civilian groups, thus affecting study results.

What is PTSD? Why do people suffer from it? Were the nurses who served in Vietnam particularly susceptible to PTSD? For the nurses in this study, PTSD was the psychological fallout of their service in Vietnam. Two central features characterized their disorder. On the one hand, the women with PTSD reexperienced the war in painful recollections, and recurrent dreams and nightmares. On the other, they also felt numb and experienced a loss of emotional reaction to the world around them. The two features coexisted in some women; others experienced them alternately in cycles. Thus, a nurse with PTSD might have high levels of reexperienced symptoms and high levels of numbness at the same time. Symptoms of PTSD included exaggerated startle response, feelings of alienation, diminished interest in activities, nightmares, disturbed sleep, guilt, difficulty concentrating, and purposeful avoidance of activities that recalled the war.[18]

California psychologist M. J. Horowitz developed a "stress response theory" to explain PTSD. Horowitz assumes that all people who survive a traumatic experience have a "completion tendency" an unconscious inclination to rethink the experience in an attempt to understand what has happened. Individuals try to connect their feelings about a traumatic event with their previous life experiences. They review memories until they understand the emotions and behaviors brought on by the traumatic event.

Horowitz refers to the characteristics of PTSD by different names, calling reexperiencing the trauma an intrusive response, and numbness about the event an avoidance response.[19] Horowitz and his colleagues developed a fifteen-item questionnaire (the Impact of Event Scale) to determine the presence of intrusive and avoidance responses of PTSD.[20] He states that people never fully complete the work of reckoning with a traumatic experience, especially an experience as intense and long as a year in a war. Even after the event no longer dominates everyday thought, waves of feeling may resurface.

The fifty nurses interviewed for this book completed Horowitz's questionnaire. They say that they agree with Horowitz: they remember well their war and are still stirred by its emotions.

Nurses commonly experienced symptoms of PTSD during their first months home. There were differences between a normal emotional recovery from Vietnam and PTSD. Nurses with

PTSD could not adequately work or relax, their symptoms were severe and taxing, and their everyday lives were affected.

Were the nurses particularly susceptible to PTSD? Researchers have identified several factors that placed people at risk of developing the disorder. They found the longer the stressful experience and the extent to which a person's life was threatened, the greater the chance of developing PTSD.[21] The women's experience in Vietnam was both prolonged and frightening, but there was another reason for their vulnerability. As a group, these nurses were altruistic. Their eagerness and sensitivity were part of their work. But what benefited patients caused the nurses to suffer. They did not stop to think about what the stresses of war might be doing to them. The motive that drove them forward, more than any other, was a passion for protecting and conserving life. The concern for preserving life begins where self-preservation ends. Dock and Stewart, in a classic history of the nursing profession, refer to this behavior as the "Mother nurse" characteristic, where tenderness and devotion to the sick and helpless came before all personal needs. The authors offered the traditional image of Florence Nightingale as an example for all nurses to follow: Nightingale was compassionate with her judgment and clear vision and fearlessly courageous in her work in the Crimean War.[22]

Nurses read Dock and Stewart's book in school. They absorbed the message and took these teachings to war. But once in Vietnam, some women came to see the inadequacy of the Dock and Stewart model. They could not ignore their own emotions. They learned to weep at pain and to lose themselves in drink as a way of maintaining their humanity. They discovered that they could not deal with all the wounded and dying day after day and remain unmoved.

Those who did try to bury their feelings never faced themselves. When they returned home, the fatigue, anxiety, anger, and other emotions they had repressed for twelve months began to surface.

One nurse, who served in Vietnam as a twenty-three-year-old lieutenant, struggled with the Nightingale image. "I felt obligated to say that my experience was not such a big deal compared to the guys over there. Now I realize that it was. I felt obligated to push it aside and say, 'Well, look, I was just a nurse and it wasn't so bad.' But it was. It took me many years before I decided that I owed it to myself, that I had the right to say it was stressful.''

The extent of PTSD among the women varied. Six women claimed they were never upset by their war memories. One of them, an army veteran, said, ''I never had a big reaction to the war. It was a matter of working it out over months rather than having a big blowup. I'm a firm believer that I went into the army to do a certain job and I had to expect it [stress] as part of the job.'' As a group, the women who reacted this way were older, married to Vietnam veterans, or involved in military careers. They lived in worlds that provided them with emotional support and stable lifestyles. They claimed not to understand the group of nurses in the study who reported major emotional reactions.

Four women found themselves depressed, alienated, and drinking because they could not forget Vietnam. They sought psychiatric counseling. Three of these women were in therapy at the time of they were interviewed.

One nurse described the difficult years. ''In 1975, and 1976, I was drinking. I didn't have many friends. I went back to school but I couldn't finish. I never took final exams because I thought I didn't deserve to graduate. I never felt I deserved anything like friends. I tried to commit suicide twice. I got tired of not liking myself and I went into therapy.'' Recently reunited with friends she served with in Vietnam, she began to sort out her memories and feelings. She and her friends talked about their war work and slowly she came to realize her guilt over the dead had been misplaced; no one was at fault.

Two of the four women who apparently suffered from PTSD were still in the military. In fact, they held high rank. All four had gone to Vietnam as young, inexperienced nurses. In contrast, the older nurses who had had more professional and personal experience before the war may have had more insight and a better perspective on their roles. Generally, those with higher levels of PTSD had been the younger, less-seasoned nurses.

Another nurse who had remained in the military began to sob at the end of her interview. ''I hurt . . . I think about all those boys. I don't know if it's a guilt I feel because I lived through it and I'm healthy and whole and here or something I've never been able to face. I never shared my pain and my grief and there is so much hurt.'' Her tears seem to encompass the same grief Vera Brittain felt in 1932 when she wrote, ''Love would seem threatened perpetually by death, and happiness appear without duration built upon shifting sands of chance.''[23]

In the years since the war, the women reported suffering other traumas—the natural progression of deaths in their families, divorces, illnesses, and the loss of their own children—but these seem to have done little to diminish their reactions to Vietnam. A nurse who served in the Army Nurse Corps said, ''I've had surgeries and lost a baby since the war. Both affected my life very much. Obviously, losing the baby was the most traumatic, but I can grieve for the baby and feel better. I've never been able to grieve about the war, so Vietnam still hurts.''

Forty-four of the nurses in this study experienced symptoms of PTSD over the years. The nurses' symptoms were brought on for reasons other than those exhibited by men who saw combat. Dewane found that medics and corpsmen also had different sources for their symptoms.[24] For example, while combat soldiers felt guilty at having survived a battle in which their friends died, corpsmen and nurses felt guilty because they thought they had not done enough to save more of the wounded.

During their first year home, twenty nurses reported feeling many intrusive symptoms of PTSD. But the emotion most frequently noted in the interviews was anger. They did not direct their anger at a specific person or object. Rather, they expressed anger at ''the war.''

Their inability to understand the reasons for the war prompted much of the anger. One women said, ''I was angry. I am angry. I still think it was a waste of young men's lives. I don't think we accomplished anything.''

''The devastation, the hopelessness, and the inability to do anything about it. You were totally impotent. It was like you were in the middle of a whirlwind trying to retain your position, let alone advance. It was so totally useless,'' said a former army nurse. There was no common foe, like Hitler or Nazism, no common idea, like ''freedom'' or democracy.'' In the end, there was no military victory, no reward for the grief.

They went to Vietnam filled with idealism and stories of

triumph from previous wars. They came home disillusioned and disquieted.

"I was angry for a long time. I don't know why I was so angry," said a nurse who chose to stay in the military. "I was angry with life. It shouldn't be this way. Now it seems stupid because I know life's not a gift, but I expected that it was." Today, these nurses say they would never blindly volunteer again. They claimed to have learned a timeless, difficult lesson in Vietnam—the reality of war is different from the dreams of youth.

"If I had to describe Vietnam, I'd use a color," said one nurse. "I'd say it was brown—a big brown smudge. Vietnam was such a waste of life. I still feel strongly about this even though so much time and so much has happened to me since [the war]. I'm still angry at the fact that it happened at all."

They directed some of their anger at "politicians who lost the war," "draft dodgers" who now enjoy the right to vote, and public treatment of male Vietnam veterans, scorned at first, then suddenly "fashionable." One women said her anger surfaced whenever she heard the expression, "blow the bastard away." "I feel like saying [to those people], 'You SOB, you have no idea what a gunshot looks like.'"

As a group, they did not take their anger to the streets or try to change government policy. They preferred to kept their feelings—along with their war experiences—to themselves. There was a sense that their anger made them different, unlike their nurse predecessors. They could not recall World War II or Korean War veteran nurses expressing anger or talking about their emotional upheavals after these wars.

The second most commonly felt symptom of PTSD was an "uncontrolled recall." Sometimes, unwarranted images interrupted everyday life. An army nurse who remained in the military said, "It's like a film. You start one frame and you dont' know where it is going. It isn't like you can check off a box. You don't know where it is going. Somebody will say something that is totally unrelated [to the war] and I'll remember something about an episode [in Vietnam] that happened. There is no conscious desire or need to dig into that stuff again." According to Horowitz, these unbidden views of the war will continue until the subject comes to terms with the event.[25]

Through the years, specific incidents brought back memories. "Saigon fell and I remember crying, 'My god, what was it all for?' " said a nurse. Pictures of the North Vietnamese in Saigon made many feel that the war and the sacrifices were in vain. The warm, heroic welcome the Iranian hostages received in 1980 was a dramatic counterpoint to the indifference of their homecomings from Vietnam. In 1983, when American forces invaded the island of Grenada, many nurses remembered the sufferings from their own war.

That same year, terrorists blew up the marine barracks in Beirut, where the servicemen were part of a United Nations peacekeeping force. Two-hundred-forty-one Americans died in that attack.[26] A navy nurse who was on duty stateside the day of the attack said the Beirut tragedy made her remember: "We were sending [medical] teams to Europe. I looked at the teams getting ready and I started to shake all over. Somebody asked me if I was okay. All I could think about was Vietnam was happening all over again."

Particular images had a powerful effect on the nurses. "I could not sit through 'The Star-Spangled Banner' without crying," said one. "I don't like to be around fatigues. Up until 1984, I could only smell blood around them," said a woman who long ago packed away her own duty uniform. Sometimes a soap or the smell of garbage will spark a memory.

Helicopters, the vehicles used to ferry Vietnam dead and wounded, became symbols of suffering. Back home, the noise or the sight of a helicopter often provoked thoughts and feelings in all the nurses in this study. The women found themselves walking to the nearest window to see where a helicopter was heading. They unconsciously found themselves identifying the type of aircraft. "It did not matter that these helicopters might be carrying business executives rather than combat troops," said one woman. Helicopters never will be thought of as civilian transportation vehicles. They will always be filled, in memory at least, with scared and bleeding young men. "I was driving up the Garden State Parkway [in New Jersey] yesterday and I saw a state police helicopter. I could not describe the feeling, but it was unmistakable. A heavy feeling," recalled a woman who recently retired after a long military career.

Nurses who visited the Vietnam Veterans Memorial in

Washington, DC, found themselves returning to the war. Looking at the granite panels engraved with the names of the missing and dead was a moving experience. Listed in chronological order in front of them were their friends and patients. Five women mentioned that seeing the recognition accorded all Vietnam veterans at the memorial finally helped them accept what had happened.

There probably will always be events and places that trigger thoughts of the war. It is unlikely that an individual ever puts their war experiences to rest. Waves of involuntary thoughts and feelings always resurface.

Nurses reported having dreams and nightmares. Men who served in Vietnam also described sleep disturbances but the content of their dreams was different.[27] The nurses' dreams were filled with patients who floated around just out of reach and hospital wards that never ended. As one woman recalled, "Some nights I don't sleep. I dream that I'm in a big building and they are handing out fatigues and all there is is Vietnam. There are no doors and I can't get out of the building and I just got there. I don't want to stay." The symbolism here seemed obvious. She involuntarily continued to reexperience the helplessness she had felt in Vietnam. Clinicians who work with war veterans report that certain techniques, ranging from relaxation exercises to psychoanalysis, effectively reduce these unsettling visions.[28]

During their first year home, sixteen nurses said they experienced the avoidance symptoms of PTSD: alienation, diminished interest in activities, and avoidance of anything that might arouse thoughts of the war. "I tried to be a normal civilian as much as I could," said a former army nurse. "I got a job, got married, got pregnant, as if I never had taken a step out of time. I wasn't numbed to the war, *mummed* is a better word."

She and others learned to avoid any thinking about the war because they feared being overwhelmed by unbearable memories. "There are just some things about Vietnam I don't want to get into. There are some very painful, futile, frustrating things I just don't want to deal with," said another woman.

While such actions protected them from unpleasantness, they also prevented these nurses from coming to understand the war. Vietnam remained unfinished and unresolved. Some evaded thinking about the war for years: "It was too difficult for me to think about it [Vietnam]. I've hardly ever shown anybody my pictures and I haven't looked at my slides for twelve years."

Another woman said that for the last fifteen years she was careful to avoid war shows or movies on television. Other nurses shunned Veterans Administrations hospitals, the Vietnam Veterans Memorial in Washington, movies, books, and news programs about the war.

Their avoidance of memories was selective. They told funny stories at cocktail parties. One woman said she lectured to herself. "I can remember standing in my apartment when something came on the TV news. I said out loud to myself, 'I will remember the people, the good times and I will forget the rest.' "

Another nurse focused on the facts about the war, but never talked about her feelings. As she said, "My feelings about feelings [from Vietnam] are frozen, they are not thawed to this day." It appeared that the instinct for self-preservation had taken over.

Their personal avoidance mirrored the attitude of society at large, particularly during the 1970s. In those early years, there was little writing, analysis, or publicity that encouraged introspection about Vietnam. With the proliferation of war-related movies and memorials a decade later, it became more difficult to escape the war. This shift may explain why only seven women currently chose to maintain their avoidance status quo. The others have gradually begun to peer into their pasts. These seven women seemed afraid to let go. One woman, who remained in the military, described her feelings: "You are supposedly a strong, adaptable, well-adjusted person. A professional. When I work in the hospital today I allow myself to feel things. But the most moving experience of my life and I can't allow myself to feel anything. You feel like if you let go you aren't going to be able to grab on again. And yet you sit there like a single solitary soul, feeling so alone and lost because you are still there."

Two years later I encountered this woman at a military base—she looked like a different person. She had lost weight and was laughing. At one point she quietly said she had begun to think and talk about her experience. "It's getting better," she said.

It was not necessary for her and the other nurses to sift through every single day in Vietnam. What they needed to do was express the feelings they had censored in order to deal with their wartime jobs. They also needed to understand that nurses were allowed to express emotions.

In this study, the number of nurses suffering from PTSD decreased over the years. During their first year home from Vietnam, most of the nurses worked in military hospitals; the images of Vietnam still were very real, and, not surprisingly, forty-four of the nurses interviewed reported intense PTSD levels at that time. For most, these symptoms decreased over the years as friends and others helped them put the war in perspective.

During subsequent years, twenty women, or forty percent of the sample, said they experienced PTSD symptoms. At the time the interviews were conducted, this number declined to twelve women or twenty-five percent. An added reason for the decline in PTSD was the change in public attitudes. In the mid-1980s, society finally acknowledged the service and sacrifice of Vietnam veterans. The nurses noted that they were able to use this positive climate to work through their feelings. They can visit the Vietnam Memorial. Through organizations, they can more easily locate friends from the war or other Vietnam veterans. In addition, it has become socially acceptable to acknowledge their involvement with the war.

The finding that one-quarter of the nurses reported symptoms of PTSD at the time of the study was comparable to the findings of the Schnaier and Paul studies on women who served in Vietnam. These results suggest that, while women had the capacity to withstand the rigors of wartime nursing, there was a need for them to express this stressful experience.

Analysis of the interviews indicated that the more intense the nurses' war experience, the higher the incidence of PTSD. That is, the greater the professional and personal strain in Vietnam, the more there was to resolve. This finding is similar to those of the research studies conducted on male Vietnam veterans. Egendorf and others found that the greater the exposure to combat (that is, the more intense the experience), the greater the level of PTSD.[29]

Prior to conducting the research interviews, I had assumed that those women who had a high level of emotional support in Vietnam would have a lower incidence of PTSD, but an examination of the interviews in this study proved that supposition wrong. Although maintaining a circle of caring friends in Vietnam was necessary for the nurses to survive the rigors of war, the memory of this circle was not enough to sustain the women after the war. Rather, it was friends back home that affected the development of PTSD. Nurses who could count on people to listen to and support them in the postwar years had lower levels of PTSD. These women, typically, had remained in the military, and while reenlistment did not guarantee emotional health, this environment provided a sense of camaraderie not found in the civilian world. Friends gave women a sense of balance or, as an air force nurse said, "the comforting feeling that I was a normal person."

One nurse in the study went through each phase of PTSD. Her experience illustrated the complexity of the syndrome. She had involuntary visions of patients and experienced panic attacks, avoidance symptoms, a bout with alcoholism, and general alienation:

After Vietnam, I thought I was going crazy, and I said to myself, "Mary [a pseudonym], drive yourself to Walter Reed [Army Hospital] and check in." I remember thinking that but I wouldn't give in. I drank a lot when I first came home and occasionally used drugs because I was trying to deal with the war. I was having nightmares. I wasn't talking to anybody. This all happened my first year home. The only time I talked about the war was when I was drinking. People stopped associating with me so I got caught up in the war by myself. It seemed that Vietnam was always with me and I couldn't escape from it. I had a severe depression that I never associated with Vietnam. I decided that it was a personal weakness on my part that I had not been able to deal with all the stuff from the war. At night, visions of these patients would come back to me. I decided there was really something wrong with me.

In 1975, I stopped drinking, joined AA [Alcoholics Anonymous], and got my life together. I thought I put Vietnam behind me. Then in 1982, I read this article on PTSD. I wanted no part of it. Yet, for some reason, I decided to go to a conference on PTSD and Vietnam. Coming back on the airplane, I was losing it. I came back on Friday and by Sunday I thought I was having a nervous breakdown. I was good at presenting myself as a healthy person. But here I was having panic attacks. If I lay down, these patients would swim around. I was having muscle twitches at work. It was more frightening than my drinking.

I told a friend of mine who was a psychiatric nurse I needed help but I wanted a female psychologist with no vested interest in Vietnam. I still thought it was me. I did not want [psychotropic] drugs. During my one and a half years in therapy, I relived some of my wartime experiences, only this time I really let myself feel. I got angry, upset, sad, and I grieved for those men. In Vietnam, I had no emotions attached to the experience. Today, I'm much better, and I found out I'm not crazy.

13

Lessons Learned from the War

If the nurses in this study were asked to draw a diagram of their lives, they most likely would sketch a straight line: the beginning of the line would represent their births and the end would be the present. The line is a continuum and represents a life filled with the usual landmarks—homes, children, husbands, friends. Like other women, they enjoy watching their children grow. At the end of the day, they are tired. There is a predictable pace to their lives.

Their Vietnam experience, however, does not fit into this rhythm or follow this straight line. The nurses would probably put the war on a small line above everything else. Vietnam was unique in their lives. Nothing before or after compared with the stresses and the rewards of serving overseas. Because of its uniqueness, the war continues to be a focal point to which their other life experiences are compared. "Nothing," said a former army nurse who lives in rural New Jersey, "can ever be the same after you've been in that environment."

Just as war has always been a crucible for men, so too is it for women. Wars are not a test of masculinity; rather, they are a crucible of humanity in which participants are given the opportunities to witness and understand extremes in human behavior. In

Vietnam, any of the nurses' illusions or naiveté disappeared in the operating rooms, on the helicopters, along the receiving wards, and in the postoperative units. Each nurse saw courage and selflessness, cruelty and cowardice. They came to know fear and vulnerability—not just in their patients but in themselves as well. The women learned they were not above the weaknesses they saw in others. Before the war, many of the nurses, because of their sheltered existence, had had a sense of security. After the war, they lost this control and discovered their own weaknesses and inadequacies: they found they were human.

The nurses who served in Vietnam returned home, like many of their fellow soldiers, with a knowledge that they had survived the worst of life's experiences. One woman, now in her early forties with a successful military career in the Army Nurse Corps Reserves and as a nursing administrator in a large city medical center, looked back on 1968 and the Tet Offensive, when she served at an evacuation hospital: "What it [the war] taught me was that I can truly do anything. Nothing can happen to me that is any better or worse. I have no fear. What can anyone possibly do to me? Send me back to Vietnam?"

This sense of confidence was new to a group of women raised and schooled to be dependent on fathers, husbands, and physicians. In Vietnam they had to be assertive and had to delegate responsibility. They had to learn to accept the consequences for any personal or professional decisions they might make. Most of all, they had to learn they were not responsible for the deaths of the young men in their care. "It was something out of my hands," said a nurse currently in the Air Force Nurse Corps Reserves who recalled the many casualties she had seen. The war forced the women to mature, to come of age.

In Vietnam there were no understanding parents, no comfortable bedrooms or dormitories. They learned to take care of themselves and their friends. They had only each other.

This bond between friends has carried over to veterans from other wars. Such bonds have traditionally been male because war is primarily a male enterprise, but the nurses became part of war's fraternity. The women deepened their relationships with their fathers and grandfathers as a result of their common war experiences.

One former army nurse, now a student at a rabbinical seminary, frequently comes into contact with Israeli soldiers who have fought more recent battles in Lebanon. She has learned about the veteran's universal sense of comradeship. "I can understand some of what the Israeli soldiers talk about. I never was in battle, but I can understand their fear. I understand, better than someone who hasn't been there [in war], the kind of stress a war puts one in. I do feel a kind of bond with them."

Political positions may differ, but the knowledge that they had survived the realities of war unites these nurses and soldiers in a special fellowship.

The Vietnam War broadened the nurses' sense of the world. One women, who had left her home state of North Dakota when she joined the army, said, "It was an educational process realizing that part of the world lives like this—the terrible poverty and the war all around them. You come from a nice family and a nice, safe environment and all of sudden nothing is safe."

Others learned to live and work with people they most likely would not have come to know elsewhere: people of different ages, religions, sexual orientations, and races. They learned tolerance.

The nurses also developed an appreciation for conveniences they once took for granted: running water, hot showers, fresh milk, fruit, and vegetables, dry clothes, and a good night's sleep. They began to value the quality of everyday life.

They came away from Vietnam changed and wiser about the toll war takes. "A piece of me got old in Vietnam and a piece of me has been an old lady ever since Vietnam, even though I was only twenty-two when I was there," said a former army nurse who now lives in Pennsylvania.

This feeling of having aged comes from losing one's sense of immortality while still young: it was impossible to spend a year working with casualties and avoid thinking about death or the fragility of existence. This sense of age was also the result of living a year under intense pressure and stress. Everyone asked something of the nurses: patients expected physical care with a soothing feminine touch; men wanted a woman to talk to and someone to remind them of home; some looked for sex while others were content with companionship; the Vietnamese children craved maternal love and the civilian adults required health care—the demands of a lifetime were compressed into twelve months.

In addition to learning the somber lessons of the war, these women became skilled in the art of nursing. One nurse, who now works with cancer patients, said, "Working in Vietnam made me feel more confident of my technical and management abilities at the same time it made me much more compassionate and caring. The war made me a better nurse. And I learned when you do a good job of taking care of patients it's very rewarding. Nursing can be very good."

These feelings were especially true for the nurses who had their first professional experiences in Vietnam. They perfected their professional skills in an atmosphere that encouraged and rewarded them. Even the more experienced nurses said that the work environment in Vietnam brought them back to their profession's origins, to the goal of providing humane, skillful care to the sick and injured. A woman who recently retired after a forty-year nursing career said, "I felt more of a nurse that year [in Vietnam] than I ever did before or since."

At the end of each interview, I asked each woman what advice they would give a young nurse about to leave for wartime duty. No one laughed or gave a glib reply like "bring lots of shampoo or hair spray." Most women thought for a moment and said they would attempt to prevent others from repeating their mistakes or encourage nurses to be more realistically prepared for war. They often spoke as if they were advising younger sisters or daughters.

The majority of the women spoke about the need to make friends who they could rely on for support. A former army nurse who had lost touch with the people she served with in Vietnam and who had not spoken about her war experience until the research interview said, "I would advise anyone going to war to talk things out with people around her. Make use of people and make good friends because camaraderie is very comforting."

The nurses in this study automatically placed themselves in the role of protectors. They still felt a responsibility to care for people younger and more vulnerable. A women who recently retired from the military said, "They [nurses] could get very discouraged after a while [in a war]. I would want them to know there are people out there who *do* care and are interested in them. They are not alone. It is important for them to know this."

The navy nurse who became unnerved watching younger nurses prepare to leave for Europe after terrorists blew up the Marine Corps barracks in Beirut in 1986 felt the same way. She watched the nurses pack their bags, then told them "to lean on one another and give the very best care they could. If they needed anything, I was back here for them."

Several said they would advise young nurses to "be fair to your emotions. If you feel down, you're down. Don't try to be something you're not." The nurses said that the label "courageous women" was a dangerous one because it implied a toughness and an ability to master emotions. "Learn you are not an iron horse," they said. "Don't be afraid of falling on your face. You can't be perfect. Pull your feelings out and examine them. Absolutely maintain your sense of humor."

They knew that maintaining a stiff exterior could result in an internal buildup of emotions that could explode into uncontrolled emotional problems such as post-traumatic stress disorder or physical ailments such as ulcers. Some nurses have paid the price for ignoring this possibility; they did not want others to do the same.

One nurse who stayed in the army nurse corps advised others "to be realistic about the things you cannot control." Another woman continued this thought, saying, "We don't always know why things happen and things don't always make sense." These nurses said that idealism and an inflated sense of self-worth have no place in war.

Another woman, a veteran of both the Korean and Vietnam Wars, wanted other nurses to realize the chaotic nature of war. "Keep your head down," she said, "and take it one day at a time." Simple advice borrowed from combat soldiers helped her survive the rigors of working with two generations of war casualties.

Not all the advice revolved around the poignant lessons of war. The women said they would encourage any nurse going to war to exploit the clinical experiences and learn as much as possible. These experiences are usually available only once in a lifetime and serve as a reward for the sacrifices nurses make when they volunteer to serve.

No one in the study wanted nurses to leave for future wars unaware of the risks. It was not until they landed in Saigon or Da Nang that most nurses realized they could lose their lives. There are names of eight dead nurses on the Vietnam Veterans Memorial in Washington.

Those women who have remained on active duty said they wanted the next generation to be prepared.[1] Their advice is given to young people sitting in classrooms in military bases across the world. War is no frolic, no game, they say.

One nurse speaks to new and potential flight nurses candidly. "I tell them we [Air Force Reserves Medical Evacuation Squadrons] will be mobilized first [in a military crisis] because of our mission. I tell them to have their things in order. To have their wills made out and if they have children to make sure they have guardians for them."

Six nurses in the study said they could not answer the question of what advice they would give. Thinking of modern technological war and terrorism, one nurse who was a retired military officer and had spent twenty-seven years watching men and women prepare for and sometimes fight wars summed up the feelings of the six when she said, "It's beyond my imagination what a war zone would be like today."

14

Conclusions

The results of my study of fifty veteran nurses support the findings of previous research conducted on nurses who served in Vietnam.[1] and echo personal accounts of nurses who served in World Wars I and II and Korea.[2] But there were three unique aspects of the Vietnam War: public antipathy toward its participants, the lack of a homecoming for its veterans, and the defeat of the South Vietnamese and the American "causes."

The inability of most of the nurses to return to Vietnam and see it at peace left the war unfinished. Some women expressed a desire to visit the orphanages, leprosariums, villages, and military bases they had known. "I'd really like to go back to Vietnam to see how the Vietnamese girl I cared for is doing as a young lady and find out what happened to my hooch, my hospital, my ward," said one army nurse.

These women want to complete their war work. They want to know about the villagers, the young orphans they clothed with outfits sent from home, the lepers with chronic disease, the hospitals they helped staff—in essence, about the place where they had finished their youth and had had some of their brightest moments.

The nurses from Vietnam have been an unrecognized group for several reasons. For one, war is considered a very masculine experience. The fact that women can survive, even thrive, during wartime, as the nurses in this study have illustrated, undermines the masculine image of war; women, nurses, do not fit the picture.

The public perception was that nurses who served in war were safe in hospitals, on ships, or in aircraft. They were not supposed to experience the raw reality of war. However, nurses, of courses, did experience "war"—not the harsh conditions of a combat soldier, but war nonetheless, with all its emotional toll. "Must women fight in combat to be considered equal?" one woman asked.

Stereotypes of nurses suggest women harder and tougher than others. Their training and their exposure to pain, sickness, and death are supposed to make them immune to mental strain. In fact, the women in this study went through a whole range of feelings during their year in Vietnam.

In her memoir about World War I Vera Brittain talks about the terrible loss and desolation she experienced during the war years. It was her wartime nursing service that propelled her toward a life as an active pacifist. Yet even this woman who had seen war's horror acknowledged an incredible sense of vigor at the front lines. "The heightened consciousness of wartime, the glory seen by the enraptured eyes of a twenty-two-year-old will be no more. . . . The world . . . has grown tame compared to that year of excitement and anguish."[3]

A nurse who served at the seventy-first Evacuation Hospital at Pleiku in 1969 echoed Brittain's sentiments: "I don't think I am ever going to find that kind of working situation again. I think I've been hunting for it for fifteen years and I've finally come to see that it's unrealistic to expect to find it again. It was a very special time in my life."

Analyzing the nurses' interviews made it clear that there also was a contradictory quality to the experience of being women in a war. The nurses were valued as professionals, yet exploited as women. They were both appreciated and used. Military leaders needed nurses to staff hospitals and care for patients but did little to accommodate the practical needs of the women. Military clothes—including protective flak jackets and helmets—did not fit. Starched white dresses and caps were particularly impractical clothing for the tropical heat or on the rolling ocean but in naval hospitals and ships and at the large third Field Hospital in Saigon white uniforms were the mandated dress code. The nurses were expected to maintain a feminine image and display feminine behavior at the same time as they treated mutilated patients. The nurses did not stop to question the inconsistencies evident in these wartime attitudes. There was so much upheaval around them, the issue of being a woman in a war zone seemed unimportant.

Many nurses chose to emphasize the positive aspects of Vietnam service. They especially recall the camaraderie they had with other military personnel. This unconscious decision to remember the worthwhile facets of Vietnam was most clear at the end of each interview when I posed the hypothetical question: would she volunteer again for duty in a war zone?

I had assumed most nurses would answer no. The opposite proved to be true. Forty-five nurses, or ninety percent of the research sample, responded affirmatively. Many of the women qualified their answers, but clearly the memory of the excitement, camaraderie, and professional challenges held sway over the grimmer aspects of wartime service.

Seven of the women said things like, "It would take me twenty minutes to get packed" or, "In a heartbeat I'd be ready."

Five nurses could not forget the stress of Vietnam. When asked whether they would serve again, they simply said no, without giving an explanation for their answers. One, however, remembered that some men did not have a choice. She recalled the patients in Vietnam and the treatment these veterans, draftees, and volunteers received at home. "I would never go back and work in a war but I would always support our youth who fought it."

At the time of the interviews, two army nurses worked in the military's rapid deployment forces. These organizations would be the first to be sent into an area of unrest or strife. Another nurse, a navy commander, was involved in outfitting a new hospital ship. For these women, the question about serving in another war was real. All three said their Vietnam experience made them particularly suited to lead others in wartime work. One women, referring to fellow officers who lack her war background, said, "I know I'll be a better head nurse than any of them."

The other thirty-five women said they would volunteer once more, but they qualified their responses. These women no longer viewed war naively or made hasty decisions.

Four nurses could not separate themselves from their roles as mothers. One responded, "Go back? Yes, if it weren't for my four children." Another woman said she would be the first one to leave for a war zone if her three children were older and did not need her any longer.

Some nurses had volunteered for war to protect their draft-eligible brothers. They knew that only one family member at a time could serve in a combat zone, and they reasoned that it was safer for someone to spend time working in a hospital or on a ship and airplane then fighting in a jungle.

Three women said they would volunteer this time to protect their children. "I have two daughters and I hope they never have to be involved in a war. I'd rather me than them go," one said.

The hesitation I noted in the voices of the other twenty-eight women was most likely absent when they volunteered for duty in Vietnam. These doubts come from experience and maturity. As middle-aged women, some face the responsibility of caring for ailing parents. One former army nurse expressed the feelings of several women who care for their parents. "I have concerns now that I didn't have at that time, but if I felt that our people were suffering and dying to the extent that I felt they were in Vietnam, yes, I'd go."

Others nurses faced the reality of their own aging. They know their stamina and endurance are no longer limitless. "War is a young people's outfit," said an officer who is near retirement age.

A few nurses were suspicious of politicians and the political motives that send men to fight. The nurses had learned to be skeptical of government policy during their service in an unpopular war. Next time, they said, they would want a clear commitment from government leaders. "Yes, I would volunteer again but it would depend on where and why the war started. I'm forty years old now. I was twenty-three when I went to Vietnam and I had stars in my eyes at that age. No more.'' Overall, however, their willingness to repeat the experience illustrated the complex and irresistible nature of war.

As a group, the women had no standard reaction to the war. Most of them lead productive, balanced lives. The war remains present, but does not consume their daily thoughts. Nine nurses in the sample continue to experience nightmares and uncontrolled images. Three others force themselves to forget the war; for them, the memories are too painful to face. They are as much victims of the Vietnam War as the male veterans who struggle with physical and mental disabilities.

Their experiences suggest that the amount of preparation for wartime nursing and the maturity of the nurse—her age, number of jobs, and years in the military prior to going overseas—may affect her ability to balance the strains and demands of war work. Those women with professional experience and confidence in their nursing skills seemed better able to deal with the demands in Vietnam than the inexperienced nurses.

Still, the professional ethos, to protect and conserve life, that guided many nurses in Vietnam may have put them at risk for developing post-traumatic stress disorder. Their regard for others took priority over self-preservation. Some nurses returned home so spent that they had little mental or physical energy left to adjust to peacetime life. Recent books articles and other media attention has raised public awareness and interest in this group of nurses.[4] More people want to hear stories and to acknowledge the work these nurses did in Vietnam.

There was no indication from the women in this study that they desired any formal salute for their war work, although individuals are working to gain federal approval for a statue honoring all female nurses, all women, who served in Vietnam.[5] None thought of themselves as heroes. They wanted to be remembered simply as women who served in war in order to help save lives. They preferred to be portrayed realistically, with all their insecurities, mistakes, and postwar adjustments. Most of all, they wanted to be thought of as skilled professionals who did their jobs well without regard to politics, either on the battlefield or at home.

I conducted the last interview of this project in my home in Montclair, New Jersey, just before Christmas 1984. The nurse I interviewed, a former army lieutenant who went on to become a midwife working in rural eastern Pennsylvania, offered to drive to my home. She had a day off work and said she would enjoy the ride through western New Jersey. I was pleased that the study would end right where it had begun, in my home. After we finished, I looked at her photo album. Then we talked about our children and our work. By ending the session that way, with talk about the present, we followed the pattern of most of the previous interviews. It was the nurses' way of telling me that they really were no different from other women.

But I came to see a difference between those women who have been to war and those who have not. There is a difference in their voices. They possess a self-confidence, and know that no future test will be as difficult as the one they had passed in Vietnam. There was no cynicism in their voices. Yes, I heard anger, sadness, and skepticism during the interviews, but these women appreciated their lives after seeing so much death. They had seen self-sacrifice and courage in Vietnam. After such witness, it was hard to be cynical.

I spent most of 1985 transcribing tapes and listening to those voices again. I think I've learned what it was like to be a military nurse in Vietnam. I think I understand the women who shared that experience.

I know now why my mother, a veteran of World War II, a Coast Guard Spar, speaks so fondly of her wartime work. She remembers the excitement and the camaraderie of being in uniform. She was young, she says, and life was simple. The nurses in this study are, in a way, my mother's kin.

As a doctoral student, I set out to write a dissertation, a monograph on wartime nursing. I wanted to record the Vietnam experience and the effect the Vietnam War had on the nurses who served there. The women I interviewed had a much more profound effect on my life than I ever would have guessed. I gained a new respect and appreciation for my profession. The nurses who served in Vietnam showed me that tenderness and compassion are not trite labels, professional clichés. They are assets, a nurse's assets. These women used those values to make an important contribution in the Vietnam War. In saving so many lives, they invested in the future. I also came to see these women as links to our past, as conduits for bringing the best of it forward. I hope their story serves as a testimony for women yet to wear a nurse's uniform, and as a lesson for the thousands of us who never have to go to war.

Appendix: Information on the Fifty Military Nurses

Information Obtained in 1983–1986 on the Fifty Nurses Who Participated in the Study

In the following table, figures for "current nursing position" do not include the three retired nurses and three women working in other fields.

Variable	Category	Frequency (N = 50)	Percentage of sample
Branch of service	Army	33	66
	Navy	14	28
	Air Force	3	6
Current military status	Active duty	12	24
	Reserve duty	15	30
	Civilian or retired officer	23	46

(Continued)

Variable	Category	Frequency (N = 50)	Percentage of sample
Current age	35–39	26	52
	40–44	15	30
	45–49	1	2
	50–55	4	8
	55 or older	4	8
Marital status	Never married	20	40
	Married	22	44
	Separated or divorced	8	16
Number of children	None	30	60
	One	4	8
	Two	6	12
	Three	7	14
	Four or more	3	6
Professional education	Nursing diploma	5	10
	Associate degree in nursing	2	4
	Bachelor's degree in nursing	11	22
	Master's degree in nursing	20	40
	Master's degree in other fields	8	16
	Doctoral degree in nursing	3	6
	Doctoral degree in other fields	1	2
Current nursing position*	Staff nurse	9	18
	Head nurse	1	2
	Nursing education faculty	4	8
	Nursing administration	20	40
	Other (clinical specialist, midwife, flight nurse, etc.)	10	20

Descriptions of the Fifty Women Interviewed

The information presented here was obtained in interviews in 1983 and 1984. Entries marked with an asterisk * were updated in 1989.

1. Interviewed 11/14/83 in New York City. Prior to the war, she held one nursing position in a stateside military hospital. As a navy nurse corps lieutenant in her early twenties, she served on the USS *Sanctuary* from March 1968 to March 1969. Assigned to work in the intensive care and surgical units. Awarded a Unit Citation. Married with two children, she accepted a commission in the navy nurse corps reserve after this interview took place.*

2. Interviewed 11/27/83 in Newark, New Jersey. Prior to the war, she had worked for less than one year in a stateside military hospital. In her early twenties she was promoted in Vietnam from lieutenant to captain in the army nurse corps. She worked at the sixty-seventh Evacuation Hospital in Qui Nhon from October 1970 to October 1971. Assigned to work in the emergency/receiving unit. Awarded the Bronze Star. Married to a Vietnam veteran, she has three children and works in community health nursing.*

3. Interviewed 12/10/83 in Norristown, Pennsylvania. Previous wartime nursing experience in the Korean conflict. Remained on active duty in the army nurse corps until 1953. Returned to active duty in 1959. In her forties she served as a major at the third Field Hospital in Saigon from April 1968 to April 1969. Assigned to work in nursing administration and on medical-surgical wards. Awarded the Bronze Star. She retired from the military with the rank of colonel.

4. Interviewed 12/10/83 in Philadelphia. She had had seven years of nursing experience prior to serving on the USS *Sanctuary* from February 1969 to February 1970. in her late twenties she was promoted from lieutenant to lieutenant commander in the navy nurse corps at the end of her Vietnam tour. Assigned to work in the multi-trauma unit. Awarded the Navy Commendation Medal. She remains on active duty at the rank of commander.

5. Interviewed 3/19/84 in Philadelphia. Prior to the war she had had six months' nursing experience. As an army nurse corps lieutenant in her early twenties, she served six months at the twelfth Evacuation Hospital in Cu Chi and six months at the twenty-fourth Evacuation Hospital in Long Binh from April 1970 to March 1971. Assigned to work in the recovery room and postoperative wards in both facilities. Resigned her commission one year after the war. Currently works as a nursing administrator in a large urban hospital.

6. Interviewed 3/21/84 in Toms River, New Jersey. Prior to the war she had had six months of nursing experience. In her early twenties she was promoted from lieutenant to captain at the end of her Vietnam tour. Assigned to the twenty-fourth Evacuation Hospital in Long Binh from April 1971 until May 1972 in the maxillofacial ward. Currently a major in the army nurse corps reserve, she is married with three children.

7. Interviewed 3/30/84 in Millburn, New Jersey. Prior to the war she had had more than ten years of military nursing experience in the army nurse corps reserve. Her reserve unit was activated for duty in Vietnam. A major in her forties, she was the nursing administrator at the seventy-fourth Field (POW) Hospital in Long Binh from September 1968 to August 1969. Awarded a Bronze Star and Unit Citation. She retired from the army nurse corps reserve with the rank of colonel.*

8. Interviewed 4/15/84 in Denville, New Jersey. Prior to the war she had had one year of nursing experience. She was married before the war and, as a lieutenant in her early twenties, she served in Cu Chi with her husband from December 1968 to November 1969. Assigned to the emergency/receiving ward. Resigned her commission one year after the war. The mother of one child, she died in February 1989 after a lengthy illness.*

9. Interviewed 4/30/84 in Bethesda, Maryland. Prior to the war she had served on active duty in the navy nurse corps from 1951 to 1954. Returned to active duty in 1960. Military tours included assignment as a navy nurse corps recruiter and overseas duty in Spain before Vietnam. As a commander in her early forties, she was assigned to the USS *Repose* from March 1968 to April 1969

and worked as a nursing administrator in the operating room. Awarded the Navy Commendation Medal. Retired with the rank of admiral. Currently married to a Vietnam veteran, she works as a consultant to veteran and military organizations.*

10. Interviewed 4/30/84 in Bethesda, Maryland. Prior to the war, she had had two years of military nursing experience. As a navy nurse corps lieutenant (jg) in her twenties, she served on the USS *Repose* from August 1966 to September 1967. Assigned to work in the intensive care, orthopedic, and postoperative units. Awarded a Unit Citation. Currently married to a Vietnam veteran, she is the mother of four children; she remains in the navy nurse corps reserve at the rank of captain and specializes in geriatric nursing.*

11. Interviewed 5/20/84 in Princeton, New Jersey. Prior to the war, she had had six months of nursing experience. As an army nurse corps lieutenant in her twenties, she served at the twelfth Evacuation Hospital from March until November 1970 and at the twenty-fourth Evacuation Hospital from November 1970 to March 1971. Assigned to work in the intensive care unit and postoperative wards. Awarded the Bronze Star. Served on active duty two years after the war. Divorced, she works in nursing administration at a large suburban hospital.

12. Interviewed 5/23/84 in Philadelphia. Prior to the war, she had had two years of nursing experience. As a navy nurse corps lieutenant in her twenties, she served at Naval Support Activity Da Nang from December 1969 to May 1970. Assigned to work in the medical wards. Awarded a Unit Commendation. Married to a Vietnam veteran, they have two children. She recently retired from active duty at the rank of commander.*

13. Interviewed 5/25/84 in Brick Town, New Jersey. Prior to the war, she had had thirteen years of military nursing experience in the navy nurse corps. As a lieutenant commander in her thirties, she was assigned to prepare the USS *Repose* for wartime service in November 1965. She remained on board and served as a nursing administrator for medical and psychiatric units from February 1966 to November 1966. Awarded a Unit Commendation.

She continued on active duty for eight years after the war and retired at the rank of commander. Currently, she works with Vietnam veterans as a psychiatric nursing specialist.*

14. Interviewed 5/31/84 in East Orange, New Jersey. Prior to the war, her only nursing experience had been as a children's camp nurse. In her early twenties she was promoted in Vietnam from lieutenant to captain in the army nurse corps. She worked at the sixty-seventh Evacuation Hospital in Qui Nhon from March 1969 to March 1970. Assigned to work in the intensive care/recovery room. She remains in the army nurse corps reserve with the rank of lieutenant colonel. Living with a Vietnam veteran, she works in hospital administration.*

15. Interviewed 6/4/84 in Bethesda, Maryland. Prior to the war, she had had two years of military nursing experience in the navy nurse corps. As a lieutenant (jg) in her twenties, she worked on the USS *Repose* from September 1967 to October 1968. Assigned to work in the postoperative thoracic ward. Awarded a Unit Commendation. She resigned her commission the same week she returned home from Vietnam. Currently married to a Vietnam veteran, she has four children and works as a faculty member at a private university where she teaches psychiatric nursing.*

16. Interviewed 6/4/84 in Bethesda, Maryland. Prior to the war, she had had thirteen months of military nursing experience. In her early twenties she was promoted from lieutenant (jg) to lieutenant in the navy nurse corps during her service on the USS *Sanctuary*. She worked in the renal dialysis unit and intensive care unit from December 1969 to December 1970. Received the Navy Achievement Award. She remains on active duty with the rank of captain. She has worked in both critical care nursing and nursing administration.*

17. Interviewed 6/5/84 in Bethesda, Maryland. Prior to the war, she had had two years of military nursing experience that included working with medical and psychiatric Vietnam casualties. As a lieutenant in her early twenties, she worked at Naval Support Activity Da Nang from February 1969 to February 1970. Assigned to the intensive care unit, she unsuccessfully tried to extend her Vietnam tour. Awarded two Unit Citations. She re-

cently married and has retired from the navy nurse corps at the rank of commander.*

18. Interviewed 6/5/84 in Bethesda, Maryland. Prior to the war, she had been on active duty in the navy nurse corps since 1951. She worked with casualties, mainly amputees, from the Korean War. A lieutenant commander, she served in Vietnam as part of an intraservice team charged with teaching surgical techniques to the Vietnamese. From February 1965 to March 1966, she worked in the Mekong Delta at Rach Gia. Awarded the Navy Commendation Medal. She retired from active duty at the rank of captain with thirty-three years of service in the navy nurse corps.*

19. Interviewed 6/5/84 in Bethesda, Maryland. Prior to her service in the war, she had had four years of military nursing experience in the operating room that included working with Vietnam casualties. As a lieutenant in her thirties, she received twenty-four hours' notice to report to Naval Support Activity Da Nang in February 1968 during the Tet Offensive. She worked as a staff nurse and administrator in the operating room until February 1969. Awarded the Navy Commendation Medal. She recently retired from active duty at the rank of captain in the navy nurse corps.*

20. Interviewed 6/6/84 in Bethesda, Maryland. Prior to the war, she had had two years of military nursing experience in the navy nurse corps. As a lieutenant in her twenties, she served on the USS *Repose* from September 1967 to September 1968. Assigned to work in the intensive care unit. Awarded a Unit Citation and the Navy Commendation Medal. Married with two children, she recently retired from active duty at the rank of commander.*

21. Interviewed 6/6/84 in Bethesda, Maryland. Prior to her service in the war, she had had three years of military nursing experience that included working with Vietnam casualties. As a lieutenant in her early twenties she served on the USS *Repose* from March 1967 to April 1968. Assigned to work in the intensive care unit, the postoperative orthopedic unit, and the ears, nose, and throat unit. Awarded a Unit Citation. She remains on active duty with the rank of captain in the navy nurse corps and works as a nursing administrator.*

22. Interviewed 6/6/84 in Bethesda, Maryland. Prior to the war, she had had four years of military nursing experience in the navy nurse corps. As a Lieutenant (jg) in her early twenties, she served on the USS *Repose* from October 1966 to October 1967. Assigned to work in the operating room, the postoperative orthopedic unit, and the ears, nose, and throat unit. Awarded a Unit Commendation. Currently on active duty with the rank of captain.*

23. Interviewed 6/8/84 in Plainfield, New Jersey. Prior to her service in the war, she had had thirteen months of military nursing experience that included working with Vietnam casualties. In Vietnam in her early twenties she was promoted from lieutenant to captain. She served at the sixty-seventh Evacuation Hospital in Qui Nhon from November 1967 to December 1968. Assigned to work in the postoperative surgical unit and orthopedic ward. She resigned her army nurse corps commission within one year of returning home. Currently married to a Vietnam veteran, she has three children and works in nursing education.

24. Interviewed 6/18/84 in New York City. Prior to the war, she had had three and one-half years of nursing experience. In her early twenties she was promoted from lieutenant to captain while in Vietnam. In Qui Nhon, she served ten months at the eighty-fifth Evacuation Hospital and two months at the sixty-seventh Evacuation Hospital from February 1968 to February 1969. Assigned to the intensive care unit/recovery room and postoperative unit at both facilities. Awarded a Bronze Star and a Unit Citation. She remains in the army nurse corps reserve with the rank of colonel. She earned a doctorate degree in nursing and works as a nursing administrator at a large urban hospital.

25. Interviewed 6/27/84 in Fairlawn, New Jersey. Prior to the war, she had two years military nursing experience in the army nurse corps. As a second lieutenant in her early twenties, she served at the twelfth Evacuation Hospital in Cu Chi from June 1969 to May 1970. Assigned to work in the emergency/receiving unit. Awarded a Bronze Star and the Army Commendation Medal. She resigned her commission within one year of returning home. Married to a veteran she met in Vietnam, she has two children. She works in the emergency room of a small rural hospital.

26. Interviewed 7/5/84 in New Windsor, New York. Prior to the war, she had had one year of nursing experience. As a lieutenant in her early twenties she served at the twenty-ninth Evacuation Hospital in Can Tho from June 1969 to July 1970. Assigned to work in the Vietnamese and medical units. Awarded the Bronze Star. Married to a Vietnam veteran, she has three children and works as a staff nurse in the emergency room of a small rural hospital.

27. Interviewed 7/12/84 at McGuire Air Force Base, New Jersey. Prior to the war, she had had more than five years of professional nursing experience, including a two-year tour on the Project Hope hospital ship in South America and West Africa. As a captain in her thirties, she began serving with the fifty-seventh Air Evacuation Squadron in 1968 and flew into Tan Son Nhut, Cam Ranh Bay, and Da Nang air fields to pick up casualties. Spent two-week periods based in Vietnam helping to prepare patients for flight. Assigned to the 1973 POW repatriation flight, Project Homecoming. Awarded the Air Force Commendation Medal. Married to a Vietnam veteran, she remains in the air force nurse corp reserve at the rank of colonel. She also continues to maintain active flight nurse status.*

28. Interviewed 7/12/84 at McGuire Air Force Base, New Jersey. Prior to the war, she had had four years of military nursing in the air force reserve and more than five years of experience in operating room nursing. As a captain she served with the tenth Air Evacuation Squadron and flew into Tan Son Nhut and Cam Ranh Bay. Assigned to "Golden Flow" flights (made up of military personnel with positive urine tests for drug use) from January 1972 to April 1972. Awarded the Philippine Cross. She remained an active flight nurse in the Air Force Nurse corp reserve and recently retired with the rank of colonel.

29. Interviewed 7/16/84 at McGuire Air Force Base, New Jersey. Prior to the war, she had had one year of nursing experience. As a lieutenant in her early twenties, she served with the 903d Air Evacuation Squadron from September 1970 to September 1971. Based in Cam Ranh Bay, she flew throughout South Vietnam, bringing casualties to various medical facilities. Awarded three

Air Medals for flying in a combat zone. She remains an active flight nurse in the air force nurse corps reserve with the rank of major. Divorced from a Vietnam veteran, she has two children and works as a nursing home administrator.*

30. Interviewed 7/29/84 in Canton, New York. Prior to the war, she had had eight months of nursing experience. In her early twenties she was promoted from lieutenant to captain while in Vietnam. She served at the seventh Surgical Hospital in Bear Cat from April 1968 to March 1969. Assigned to work in the emergency, recovery room, and postoperative units. Resigned her army nurse corps commission within one year of returning home. Married to a Vietnam veteran, she has four children and works as a psychiatric counselor to Vietnam veterans. She is active in women veterans' organizations.*

31. Interviewed 8/3/84 in Newark, Delaware. Prior to the war, she had had one year of nursing experience. As a lieutenant in her early twenties, she served at the eighth Field Hospital in Nha Trang for six months, then transferred to the ninety-fifth Evacuation Hospital in Da Nang for the remaining six months of her tour, from May 1968 to May 1969. Assigned to work in emergency/receiving at the eighth Field Hospital and in orthopedic and medical units at the ninety-fifth Evacuation Hospital. Awarded the Army Commendation Medal. Remains in the army nurse corps reserve with the rank of major. Married, with two children, she is completing doctoral work in the field of geriatrics.

32. Interviewed 8/6/84 in Upper Montclair, New Jersey. Prior to the war, she had had less than one year of nursing experience. As a lieutenant in her early twenties, she served at the ninety-fifth Evacuation Hospital from February 1970 to February 1971. Assigned to work in intensive care and postoperative surgical units. Remains in the army nurse corps reserve with the rank of major. Married with two children, she works in critical care nursing.*

33. Interviewed 8/28/84 in Mt. Laurel, New Jersey. Prior to the war, she had had one year of army nurse corp experience that included working with Vietnam casualties. As a captain in her twenties, she served at the eighty-fifth Evacuation Hospital in Qui Nhon from April 1968 to November 1968. Assigned to work

in the intensive care/recovery room unit. Remains in the army nurse corps with the rank of major. She works in nursing administration.**

34. Interviewed 8/30/84 in Wharton, New Jersey. Prior to the war, she had had two years of military nursing experience that included working with Vietnam casualties. In her early twenties she was promoted from second to first lieutenant in the army nurse corps while in Vietnam. She served at the ninety-first Evacuation Hospital in Cu Lai, from September 1970 to September 1971. Assigned to work in intensive care/recovery room and postoperative surgical units. Awarded the Army Commendation Medal. Within six weeks of returning home, resigned her commission and married a veteran she met in Vietnam. The mother of two children, she works as a staff nurse on a medical-surgical unit of a community hospital.

35. Interviewed 9/21/84 in Somerville, NJ. Prior to the war, she had had less than one year of army nurse corps experience that included working with Vietnam casualties. As a lieutenant in her early twenties, she served at the third Surgical Hospital at Can Tho from August 1969 to August 1970. Assigned to work in the intensive care/recovery room unit. Awarded the Bronze Star. Resigned her commission within one year of returning home. Divorced from a Vietnam veteran, she works as an administrator of a geriatric center.*

36. Interviewed 9/26/84 in Neubrooke, West Germany (interview conducted by a research assistant). Prior to the war, she had had one year of army nurse corps experience. As a captain in her early twenties, she served at the twenty-seventh Surgical Hospital in Chu Lai from April 1967 to April 1968. Assigned to work in the recovery room. Awarded the Bronze Star. She resigned her commission but returned to the army nurse corps within her first year home. She remains on active duty with the rank of lieutenant colonel, and she is involved in nursing management.

37. Interviewed 10/1/84 in New York City. Prior to the war, she had had less than one year of army nurse corps experience. In her early twenties she was promoted from second to first lieutenant while in Vietnam. She served at the twenty-fourth Evacuation

Hospital in Long Binh and transferred to the twenty-ninth Evacuation Hospital in Can Tho from April 1968 to April 1969. Assigned to work in the orthopedic and Vietnamese units. Awarded the Army Commendation Medal. Resigned her commission within one year of returning home. A former student at a rabbinical school, she is a staff nurse in an urban hospital and a graduate student in psychiatric nursing.*

38. Interviewed 10/10/84 in Lansdale, Pennsylvania. Prior to the war, she had had one year of military nursing experience that included working with Vietnam casualties. As an army nurse corps lieutenant in her early twenties, she served at the sixty-seventh Evacuation Hospital in Qui Nhon from February 1969 to February 1970. Assigned to work in the emergency/receiving unit. Awarded a commendation from the Republic of Korea hospital administrators. Resigned her commission within one year of returning home. Divorced from a Vietnam veteran, she is the mother of three children and works as a supervisor in a rehabilitation center.

39. Interviewed 10/12/84 in West Springfield, Massachusetts. Prior to the war, she had had less than one year of military experience, which included working with Vietnam casualties. As a lieutenant in her early twenties, she served at the ninety-fifth Evacuation Hospital in Da Nang from October 1969 to October 1970. Assigned to work in the intensive care, postoperative, and civilian units. Awarded a Bronze Star and a Purple Heart Medal for injuries received from a POW patient. Resigned her army nurse corps commission within one year of returning home. Divorced from a Vietnam veteran, she specializes in critical care nursing education.

40. Interviewed 10/12/84 in Glastonbury, Connecticut. Prior to the war, she had had less than one year of nursing experience. As a second lieutenant in her early twenties, she served at the twenty-fourth Evacuation Hospital in Long Binh from July 1970 to July 1971. Assigned to work in the neurosurgical intensive care unit. She resigned her army nurse corps commission within one year of returning home. A nurse practitioner in women's health, she works for a state health department.*

41. Interviewed 10/29/84 in Whiting, New Jersey. Prior to the war, she had had less than one year of nursing experience. As a 2d lieutenant in her early twenties, she served at the third Field Hospital in Saigon from February 1969 to February 1970. Assigned to work in the orthopedic unit. Awarded the Army Commendation Medal. She resigned her army nurse corps commission within one year of returning home. Married and the mother of two children, she works in community health nursing.*

42. Interviewed 11/2/84 in Philadelphia, Pennsylvania. Prior to the war, she had had one year of military nursing experience that included working with Vietnam casualties. In her early twenties, she was promoted from lieutenant to captain while in Vietnam. She served at the ninety-first Evacuation Hospital in Cu Lai from June 1971 to November 1971 and at the twenty-fourth Evacuation Hospital in Long Binh from November 1971 to April 1972. Assigned to work in the medical unit and intensive care unit at the ninety-first Evacuation Hospital and in the orthopedic and maxillofacial unit at the twenty-fourth Evacuation Hospital. Awarded the Army Commendation medal. Remains in the army nurse corps reserve with the rank of major. Married with three children, she works in nursing administration.

43. Interviewed 11/2/84 in Philadelphia, Pennsylvania. Prior to the war, she had had two years of military nursing experience that included working with Vietnam casualties. As a captain in her early twenties, she served in Phu Bai at the twenty-second Surgical Hospital from May to August 1969 and at the eighty-fifth Evacuation Hospital from August 1969 to May 1970. Assigned to work in the emergency/receiving unit at the twenty-second Surgical Hospital and in emergency/receiving, intensive care/recovery room, and postoperative surgical units at the eighty-fifth Evacuation Hospital. Awarded a Unit Citation. She resigned her army nurse corps commission within one year of returning home. Three of her brothers are Vietnam veterans. Works as a staff nurse in critical care nursing.

44. Interviewed 11/9/84 in Washington, DC. Prior to the war, she had had ten years of military nursing experience, including an

overseas tour. As a major in her thirties, she served at the thirty-sixth Evacuation Hospital in Vung Tau from June 1967 to December 1967 and at the sixth Convalescent Center from January 1968 to June 1968. Assigned to work in nursing administration at both facilities. Awarded a Bronze Star. Remained on active duty in the army nurse corps after the war in nursing administration. She recently retired from the military.*

45. Interviewed 11/9/84 in Gaithersberg, Maryland. Prior to the war, she had had three years of military nursing experience. As a captain in her twenties, she served at the twelfth Evacuation Hospital in Cu Chi and at the twenty-fourth Evacuation Hospital in Long Binh from June 1969 to May 1970. Assigned to the emergency/receiving ward in both facilities. Ten days before she was scheduled to return home, she became ill with pneumonia, dysentery, and obstructed biliary ducts, and had to be air-evacuated to Japan for treatment. Awarded an Army Commendation Medal and a Bronze Star. Remained on active duty two years after the war and resigned her army nurse corps commission. Works in a private management corporation.

46. Interviewed 11/10/84 in Washington, DC. Prior to the war, she had had one year of professional nursing experience that included working with Vietnam casualties. As a second lieutenant in her early twenties, she served at the seventy-first Evacuation Hospital in Pleiku from January 1969 to January 1970. Assigned to the intensive care/recovery room unit. Awarded a Bronze Star. Resigned her army nurse corps commission within one year of returning home. Works in nursing administration at a large medical center.*

47. Interviewed 11/10/84 in Washington, DC. Prior to the war, she had had less than one year of professional nursing experience. As a lieutenant in the army nurse corps, she served at the twenty-fourth Evacuation Hospital from January to August 1969 and at the seventy-first Evacuation Hospital in Pleiku from August to December 1969. Assigned to work in the neurosurgical intensive care unit at the twenty-fourth Evacuation Hospital and in the intensive care/recovery room unit at the seventy-first Evacuation Hospital. Awarded the Army Commendation Medal.

After the war, she transferred to the air force nurse corps reserve and became a flight nurse with the rank of major. She remains a reserve officer.*

48. Interviewed 11/11/84 in Washington, DC. Prior to the war, she had had less than one year of professional nursing experience that included working with Vietnam casualties. As a lieutenant in her early twenties, she served at the seventy-first Evacuation Hospital in Pleiku from April 1969 to March 1970. Assigned to work in the medical unit and postoperative surgical unit. Awarded the Bronze Star. Resigned her army nurse corps commission within two years of returning home. Active in Vietnam veterans organizations, she works as an infection control nurse at a large medical center.*

49. Interviewed 11/20/84 in New York City. Prior to the war, she had had less than one year of professional nursing experience that included working with Vietnam casualties. In her early twenties she was promoted from lieutenant to captain while in Vietnam. She served at the third Field Hospital in Saigon from June 1969 to June 1970. Assigned to work in the operating room. Awarded the Bronze Star. She remained in the army nurse corps reserve with the rank of lieutenant colonel. She recently returned to teaching in a nursing program after having worked in business positions. Married to a Vietnam veteran.*

50. Interviewed 12/19/84 in Upper Montclair, New Jersey. Prior to the war, she had had one year of professional nursing experience that included working with Vietnam casualties. As a lieutenant in her early twenties, she served at the seventy-first Evacuation Hospital from May 1970 to December 1970 and at the eighty-fifth Evacuation Hospital from January 1971 to June 1971. Assigned to work in the intensive care unit at both facilities. She resigned her army nurse corp commission within one year of returning home. Married to a Vietnam veteran, she is the mother of one child and works as a nurse midwife in a rural area.

Notes

Introduction

1. "Nurses Dispute and Defend Memoir on Life in Vietnam War" (1985, February 12), *New York Times,* p.20.
2. Vale, J. (1983), personal communication.
3. Brigadier General C. L. Slewitzke, USA, NC (1983, November 10), personal communication.
4. "Women Vets Profiled in New VA Study" (1985, October), *VVA Veteran* 5, p.6.
5. P. Theiler (1984, November/December), "A Vietnam Aftermath: The Untold Story of Women and Agent Orange," *Common Cause Magazine,* pp.29–34. S. K. Rice-Grant (1986), "Does Anyone Care: About the Health Problems of Women Who Served in Vietnam," unpublished master's thesis, California State University, Sacramento.

Chapter 1: Volunteering for the Vietnam War

1. L. Harris (1980), *Myths and Realities: A Study of Attitudes Toward Vietnam Era Veterans* (Washington, DC: U.S. Government Printing Office), p.4.

2. H. Wells (1943), *Cherry Ames: Student Nurse* (New York: Grosset and Dunlap), H. Wells (1944), *Cherry Ames: Army Nurse* (New York: Grosset and Dunlap).

3. American Nurses' Association (1967), *Facts About Nursing: A Statistical Summary—1967 Edition* (New York: American Nurses Association), p. 54.

4. "American Nurses' Association's First Position on Education in Nursing" (1966), *American Journal of Nursing* 66, 515–17.

5. M. E. Frank and R. V. Piemonte (1985), "The Army Nurse Corps: A Decade of Change," *American Journal of Nursing* 85, 985–88. P. A. Kalisch and B. J. Kalisch (1986), *The Advance of American Nursing,* 2nd edition (Boston: Little, Brown), pp. 680–81.

6. J. Holm (1982), *Women in the Military: An Unfinished Revolution* (Novato, CA: Presidio Press), pp. 70–76; 85.

7. C. Gilligan (1983), *In a Different Voice: Psychological Theory and Women's Development* (Cambridge, MA: Harvard University Press), pp. 5–23.

8. Information obtained from study interviews.

Chapter 2: Arriving in Vietnam

1. S. Neel (1973), *Medical Support of the U.S. Army in Vietnam, 1965–1970,* Department of the Army Publication No. 008-029-00088-1 (Washington, DC: U.S. Government Printing Office).

2. Similar routines are described in following books and articles: D. Freedman and J. N. Rhoads (1897), *Nurses in Vietnam: The Forgotten Warriors* (Austin, TX: Texas Monthly Press); D. Kirk (1965), "It was 2:00 A.M. Saigon Time," *American Journal of Nursing* 65, 77–79. B. McKay (1968), "Civilian Assignment," *American Journal of Nursing* 68, 336–38. S. McVicker (1985), "Invisible Veterans: The Women Who Served in Vietnam," *Journal of Psychosocial Nursing* 23, 12–19. K. Marshall (1987), *In the Combat Zone: An Oral History of American Women in Vietnam* (Boston: Little, Brown). K. Walker (1985), *A Piece of My Heart: The Stories of 26 American Women Who served in Vietnam* (Novato, CA: Presidio Press).

3. Medical civilian action patrols were also described in R. K., Tamerious (1988), "Viet Nam—A Legacy of Healing," *California Nursing Review* 10(5), 14–17, 34–38, 44–48. L. Van Devanter and C. Morgan (1983) *Home Before Morning: The Story of an Army Nurse in Vietnam* (New York: Beaufort).

4. C. R. Kneisl and S. W. Ames (1986), *Adult Health Nursing: A Biopsychosocial Approach* (Menlo Park, CA: Addison-Wesley), pp. 1217–18.

Chapter 3: The Professional Strains and Moral Dilemmas of Nursing in Vietnam

1. L. Harris (1980), *Myths and Realities: A Study of Attitudes Toward Vietnam Era Veterans* (Washington, DC: U.S. Government Printing Office), pp.3–4. "What Vietnam did to us," (1981, December 14), *Newsweek,* p.47. J. Holm (1982), *Women in the Military: An Unfinished Revolution* (Novato, CA: Presidio Press), p. 322.

3. F. Shea (1983, January–February). "Stress of Caring for Combat Casualties," *U.S. Navy Medicine,* 4–7.

4. B. G. McCaughey and J. Garrick, "Naval Support Activity Hospital Da Nang Combat Casualty Deaths January to June 1968," *Military Medicine* 152, 284–89.

5. First-person stories about mass casualty situations in American military hospitals in Vietnam are found in most writings on nurses who served in the war, such as the references listed below: D. Freedman (1984, August 19), "Women at War," *San Antonio Light,* 15–23. M. MacPherson (1984, June), "Vietnam Nurses: These are the Women Who Went to War," *Ms. Magazine,* 52–55, 104–105. C. Mithers (1984, May 29), "Picking Up the Pieces," *Village Voice,* 21–23, 42. J. D. Odom (1986), "The Vietnam Nurses Can't Forget," *American Journal of Nursing* 86, 1035–37. L. Spooner Schwartz (1988), "Women and the Vietnam Experience," *Image: Journal of Nursing Scholarship* 19, 168–73. L. Van Devanter and C. Morgan (1983), *Home Before Morning: The Story of an Army Nurse in Vietnam* (New York: Beaufort).

6. A description of triage from a physician's point of view can be found in R. J. Glasser (1971). *365 Days* (New York: Braziller).

7. J. M. Strange (1987), *Shock Trauma Care Plans* (Spring House, PA: Springhouse, p. 376.

8. J. G. Gray (1970), *The Warriors: Reflections on Men in Battle* (New York: Harper & Row), pp. 155–202.

9. J. I. Walker (1981), "The Psychological Problems of Vietnam Veterans," *JAMA,* 246, 781–82. A. S. Blank (1982), "The Stresses of War: The Example of Vietnam," in L. Goldberger and S. Breznitz (eds.), *Handbook of Stress: Theoretical and Clinical Aspects* (New York: Free Press), pp. 633–35.

10. L. L. Dock and I. M. Stewart (1932), *A Short History of Nursing: From the Earliest Times to the Present Day,* 3rd edition (New York: Putnam). S. Reverby (1987), *Ordered to Care: The Dilemma of American Nursing* (New York: Cambridge University Press).

Chapter 4: The Rewards of Wartime Nursing in Vietnam

1. J. Holm (1982), *Women in the Military: An Unfinished Revolution* (Novato, CA: Presidio Press), p.322.

2. P. A. Kalisch and B. J. Kalisch (1986), *The Advance of American Nursing,* 2nd edition (Boston: Little, Brown), p. 695.

3. C. R. Kneisl and S. W. Ames (1986), *Adult Health Nursing: A Biopsychosocial Approach* (Menlo Park, CA: Addison-Wesley), p.1714.

4. Ibid., p. 1128.

5. E. Durr (1987, January 19), "Vietnam Experience Shaped Nurse's Life," *Watertown Daily Times,* 9.

6. J. Holm, op. cit, pp. 73–74.

7. A. S. Blank (1982), "The Stresses of War: The Example of Vietnam," in L. Goldberger and S. Breznitz (eds.), *Handbook of Stress: Theoretical and Clinical Aspects* (New York: Free Press), pp. 633–35.

Chapter 5: Personal Experiences in Vietnam

1. M. J. Horowitz (1986), *Stress Response Syndromes,* 2d edition (New York: Aronson), pp. 85–86.

2. R. M. Scurfield (1985), "Post-Trauma Stress Assessment and Treatment: Overview and Formulations," in C. Figley (ed.), *Trauma and Its Wake: The Study and Treatment of Post-Traumatic Stress Disorder* (New York: Brunner/Mazel, pp. 245–46.

3. D. Spelts (1986), "Nurses Who Served—And Who Did Not Return," *American Journal of Nursing* 86,1037–39. "Army Loses Doctor and Two Nurses in Vietnam" (1966, February 28), News release from Office of the Surgeon General, U.S. Army, Technical Liaison Division, Washington, DC "Army Nurse Awarded DAR Medal Posthumously," (1970, April 27), News release from Office of the Surgeon General, U.S. Army, Technical Liaison Division, Washington, DC "Army Nurse Killed by Enemy Rocket," (1969, June 23), *Army Reporter,* 1. "First Nurse Killed in Action in Vietnam" (1969, June 13), News release from Office of the Surgeon General, U.S. Army, Technical Liaison Division, Washington, DC. B. Fisher (1983, May 29). "The Nurses Who Died in Vietnam," *Fort Worth Star–Telegram,* D1, D5. S. Neel (1973), "Medical Support of the U.S. Army in Vietnam, 1965–1970," Department of the Army Publication No. 008-029-00088-1 (Washington, DC: U.S. Government Printing Office, pp.144–45. T. R. Strum (1977, May), "By Death Undaunted," *Airman,* pp. 25–30.

4. Biographical data on nurses killed in Vietnam obtained from files at the U.S. Army Center for Military History, Special History Branch, Army Nurse Corps historical files.

5. C. Woodham-Smith (1951), *Florence Nightingale: 1820–1910* (New York: McGraw-Hill), p. 231.

6. S. Reverby (1987), *Ordered to Care: The Dilemma of American Nursing* (New York: Cambridge University Press), pp. 49–51.

7. "Drug use among American medical personnel is described in A. Santoli (1981), *Everything We Had* (New York: Random House), pp. 145–46; and L. Van Devanter and C. Morgan (1983), *Home Before Morning: The Story of an Army Nurse in Vietnam* (New York: Beaufort), p. 180. R. F. Laufer, T. Yager, E. Frey-Wouters, and J. Donnellan (1981), "Post-War Trauma: Social and Psychological Problems of Vietnam Veterans in the Aftermath of the Vietnam War," in A. Egendorf, C. Kadushin, R. Laufer, G. Rothbart, and L. Sloan (eds.), *Legacies of Vietnam: Comparative Adjustments of Veterans and Their Peers,* Report to the 97th Congress, First Session, House Committee Print Number 14, pp. 370–71.

Chapter 6: The Status of Female Military Nurses in Vietnam

1. "Women Vets Profiled in New VA Study" (1985, October), *VVA Veteran* 5, 6. L. Harris (1980), *Myths and Realities: A Study of Attitudes Toward Vietnam Era Veterans* (Washington D.C.: U.S. Government Printing Office), p. 4.

2. E. A. Paul (1985), "Wounded Healers: A Summary of the Vietnam Nurses Veterans Project," *Military Medicine* 150, 574.

3. "Much Too Macho: Sexist Treatment in the Navy and Marines" (1987, September, 28), *Time* 130, 28.

4. J. G. Gray (1970), *The Warriors: Reflections on Men in Battle* (New York: Harper & Row), pp.70–114. The romantic experiences of a World War I American nurse in Europe are told in *War Nurse: The True Story of a Woman Who Lived, Loved and Suffered on the Western Front* (1930) (New York: Cosmopolitan Book Corporation).

5. P. A. Kalisch and B. J. Kalisch (1987), *The Changing Image of the Nurse* (Menlo Park, CA: Addison-Wesley), pp. 13–14, 156–57.

6. J. Holm (1982), *Women in the Military: An Unfinished Revolution* (Novato, CA: Presidio), pp. 70–71.

7. Kalisch and Kalisch, op. cit, pp. 161–62.

Chapter 7: Different Experiences in the Army, Navy, and Air Force Nurse Corps

1. Army nurses talked about their living and working conditions in the following books: K. Marshall (1987), *In the Combat Zone: An Oral History of American Women in Vietnam* (Boston: Little, Brown). S. Saywell (1985), *Women in War: First-Hand Accounts from World War II to El Salvador* (New York: Viking). L. Van Devanter and C. Morgan (1983), *Home Before Morning: The Story of an Army Nurse in*

Vietnam (New York: Beaufort). K. Walker (1985), *A Piece of my Heart: The Stories of 26 American Women Who Served in Vietnam* (Novato, CA: Presidio Press).

2. Another incident involving Miss America and military nurses is described in M. Baker (1981), *Nam.* (New York: Quill), pp.99–100.

3. Other army nurses detailed enemy attacks in D. Elvenstar (1980, December 14), "Mary Comes Marching Home," *California Living, Los Angeles Herald Examiner*, pp. 5–10, 21; S. McVicker (1987), "Vietnam," *NSNA/Imprint* 34 42–45. L. Spooner Schwartz (1988), "Women and the Vietnam experience," *Image: Journal of Nursing Scholarship* 19 168–73.

4. Another navy nurse who served at NSA Da Nang described enemy attacks at the hospital in K. Walker (1985), op. cit., pp.203–217.

5. A Stryker frame is a bed used to immobilize patients. It consists of two metal frames on which canvas is stretched. When patients are being turned over, they are sandwiched between the two frames so that they cannot move. See C. R. Kneisl and S. W. Ames (1986), *Adult Health Nursing, A Biopsychosocial Approach* (Menlo Park, CA: Addison-Wesley, p.1201.

6. Brigadier General S. W. Wells USAF, NC (Ret.) (1989, April 5), personal communication.

7. Three air force nurses talked about their Vietnam experiences in K. Marshall (1987). *In the Combat Zone: An Oral History of American Women in Vietnam* (Boston: Little, Brown), pp. 28–34, 92–102, 158–69.

8. C. Hudak, B. Gallo, and T. Lohr, *Critical Care Nursing,* 4th edition (Philadelphia: Lippincott, 1986), pp. 264–66.

9. The dangers of flying medical evacuation flights were also described in T. R. Sturm (1977, May), "By Death Undaunted," *Airman,* 25–30. See also K. Walker (1983, September 15), "The Forgotten Vets," *San Francisco Sunday Examiner & Chronicle,* 8, 10.

Chapter 8: Factors Associated with the Year the Nurse Served in Vietnam

1. A. D. Horne (ed.), (1981), *The Wounded Generation: America After Vietnam* (Englewood Cliffs, NJ: Prentice-Hall), pp.15–29.

2. F. Fitzgerald (1972), *Fire in the Lake: The Vietnamese and the Americans in Vietnam* (Boston: Atlantic/Little, Brown), pp.369–73.

3. S. Karnow (1983), *Vietnam: A History* (New York: Viking Press, pp. 415–16.

4. Ibid., pp. 682–83.

5. B. Edelman (ed.) (1986), *Dear America: Letters Home from Vietnam* (New York: Pocket Books), pp.203–33.

6. S. Karnow (1983), *Vietnam: A History* (New York: Viking Press), pp. 523–45.

7. D. Williams (1985), *To the Angels* (San Francisco: Denson Press). M. Ullom (n.d.), *The Philippine Assignment: Some Aspects of the Army Nurse Corps in the Philippine Islands 1940–1945,* unpublished manuscript, Department of the Army, Center of Military History, Washington, DC.

8. C. Dougan and S. Lipsman (1984), *The Vietnam Experience: A Nation Divided* (Boston: Boston Publishing Company).

9. A. D. Horne (ed.), op. cit., p. 77. S. Karnow (1983), *Vietnam: A History* (New York: Viking Press), pp. 238–39, 690.

10. M. Mac Pherson (1985), *Long Time Passing: Vietnam and the Haunted Generation* (New York: Doubleday), p. 466.

11. A. D. Horne (ed.), op. cit., pp. 167–82. A. Santoli (1981), *Everything we had* (New York: Random House, 1981), pp. 153–59.

12. R. J. Lifton (1973), *Home from the War* (New York: Simon and Schuster), pp. 125–26, 171–77.

13. M. Mac Pherson, op. cit., pp. 572–76.

14. S. Karnow op. cit., pp. 685–85.

15. Ibid., p. 655.

Chapter 9: Leaving Vietnam

1. J. Haber, A. Leach, S. Schudy and B. Sideleau (1982), *Comprehensive Psychiatric Nursing,* 2nd edition (New York: McGraw-Hill), p. 269.

2. Ibid., pp. 269–74.

3. B. Edelman (ed.) (1986), *Dear America: Letters Home from Vietnam* (New York: Pocket Books), pp. 235–74.

4. B. McBryde (1979), *A Nurse's War* (New York: Universe Books), pp. 82–89.

5. *Decorations and Awards* (1984, April) Army regulations 672-5-2 July 1967 and 672-5-1 (Washington DC: U.S. Government Printing Office).

6. C. Dougan and S. Weiss (1984), *The Vietnam Experience: Nineteen Sixty-Eight* (Boston: Boston Publishing Company).

Chapter 10: Homecoming

1. C. Dougan and S. Lipsman (1984), *The Vietnam Experience: A Nation Divided* (Boston: Boston Publishing Company), p. 100

2. R. H. Stretch, J. D. Vail and J. P. Mahoney (1985), "Post-traumatic Stress Disorder Among Army Nurse Corps Vietnam veterans," *Journal of Consulting and Clinical Psychology,* 53, 704–08.

3. A. M. Schlesinger (ed.) (1983), *The Almanac of American History* (New York: Putnam), pp.445, 457, 460, 470.

4. T. Archard (1945), *G.I. Nightingale: The story of an American Army Nurse* (New York: W. W. Norton), p.181.

5. R. J. Lifton (1973), *Home from the War* (New York: Simon and Schuster), pp.157–58.

Chapter 11: The Years Since the War

1. J. Lynaugh and C. Fagin (1988, Winter), Nursing Comes of Age," *Image: Journal of Nursing Scholarship* 20, 181–90.

2. M. R. Higonnet and P. L. R. Higonnet (1987), "The Double Helix," in M. R. Higonnet, J. Jenson, S. Michel, and M. C. Weitz (eds.), *Behind the Lines: Gender and the Two World Wars* (New Haven, CT: Yale University Press), pp. 31–51.

3. Air Force nurses speak about teaching wartime procedures in B. Hoey (1984, April), "When Nurses Go to 'War'," *Airman,* 25–30.

4. United States Department of Health and Human Services (1986), *Report on Nursing. Fifth Report to the President and Congress on the Status of Health Personnel in the U.S.,* DHHS publication no. 0906804 (Washington DC: U.S. Government Printing Office).

5. C. Dougan and S. Lipsman (1984), *The Vietnam Experience: A Nation Divided* (Boston: Boston Publishing Company), pp. 177–79.

6. M. Rustad (1982), *Women in Khaki: The American Enlisted Woman* (New York: Praeger), pp.138–80.

7. A. Egendorf, C. Kadushin, R. Laufer, G. Rothbart, and L. Sloan (1981, March), "Overview of the Report," in *Legacies of Vietnam: Comparative Adjustments of Veterans and Their Peers* (report to the 97th Congress, first session), House Committee Print Number 14.

8. L. Harris (1980), *Myths and Realities: A Study of Attitudes Toward Vietnam Era Veterans* (Washington, DC: U.S. Government Printing Office).

9. Ibid.

10. E. Hess (1986, July 15), "Statue of limitation? " *Village Voice,* p.74. B. Bowers (1987, November 9), "Women Vets Fighting to Keep Monument Hope Alive," *Plainfield Courier News,* p.1. "Vietnam Veteran Nurses Remember Their Past" (1985), *American Journal of Nursing* 85, 1293. *Nurse: Vietnam Veterans Memorial Project* (1983), brochure available from Vietnam Nurse Memorial Project, 511 Eleventh Avenue South, Box 45, Minneapolis, MN 55415.

Chapter 12: Coming to Terms with the War:
Post-Traumatic Stress Disorder

1. S. Neel (1973), "Medical Support of the U.S. Army in Vietnam, 1965–1970," Department of the Army Publication No. 008-029-00088-1 (Washington, DC: U.S. Government Printing Office), p. 144.

2. V. Brittain (1933, reprinted 1978), *Testament of Youth* (London: Virago Books), pp.496–97.

3. American Psychiatric Association (1980), *Diagnostic and Statistical Manual of Mental Disorders* 3d ed, (Washington, DC: APA., p.380.

4. R. J. Daly (1983), "Samuel Pepys and Post-Traumatic Stress Disorder," *British Journal of Psychiatry* 143, 64–68.

5. J. Breuer and S. Freud (1955), *Studies in Hysteria,* standard edition (London: Hogarth Press, originally published 1895).

6. C. S. Myers (1940), *Shell Shock in France 1914–1918* (Cambridge: Cambridge University Press).

7. W. C. Menninger (1947), "Psychiatric Experience in the War, 1941–1946," *American Journal of Psychiatry* 103, 577–86.

8. R. R. Grinker and J. P. Spiegel (1945), *Men Under Stress* (Philadelphia: Blakiston).

9. H. C. Archibald, D. M. Long, and C. Miller (1962), "Gross Stress Reaction in Combat: A 15-year Follow-Up, *American Journal of Psychiatry* 119, 317–21. A. Kardiner and H. Speigel (1947), *War, Stress, and Neurotic Illness* (New York: Hoeber). F. W. Mott (1919), *War neuroses and shell shock* (London: Oxford Medical Publications.

10. R. J. Lifton (1968), *Death in Life* (New York: Random House). W. G. Neiderland (1964), "Psychiatric Disorders Among Persecution Victims: A Contribution to the Understanding of Concentration Camp Pathology and Its After Effects," *Journal of Nervous and Mental Disease* 139, pp. 458–74. E. Lindemann (1944), "Symptomatology and Management of Acute Grief," *American Journal of Psychiatry* 101, 141–48.

11. M. J. Horowitz and G. Solomon (1975), "Prediction of Delayed Stress Response Syndrome in Vietnam Veterans," *Journal of Social Issues* 31, 67.

12. A. Egendorf et al., op. cit. "Overview of the Report." C. R. Figley (ed.), (1978), *Stress Disorders Among Vietnam Veterans: Theory, Research, and Treatment* (New York: Brunner/Mazel. E. P. Nace, C. P. O'Brien, J. Mintz, N. Ream, and A. Meyers (1978), "Adjustment Among Vietnam Veteran Drug Users Two Years Post-Service," in C. R. Figley (ed.), op. cit. R. Strayer and L. Ellenhorn (1973), "Vietnam Veterans: A Study Exploring Adjustment Patterns and Attitudes," *Journal of Social Issues* 31, 81–94. J. P. Wilson (1980), "Conflict, Stress and Growth: The Effects of War on Psychological Development

Among Vietnam Veterans," in C. R. Figley and S. Leventman (eds.), *Strangers at Home: Vietnam Veterans Since the war* (New York: Praeger).

13. J. Nordheimer (1971, May 26), "Medal of Honor Winner Dies," *New York Times,* 1.

14. T. Egan (1989, January 24), "Veterans Returning to Vietnam End a Haunting," *New York Times,* 12.

15. American Psychiatric Association, op. cit., p. 380.

16. J. Schnaier (1982), "Women Vietnam Veterans and Their Mental Health Adjustment: A Study of Their Experience and Post-Traumatic stress," unpublished master's thesis, University of Maryland. E. Paul and J. O'Neill, (1986), "American Nurses in Vietnam: Stressors and Aftereffects," *American Journal of Nursing* 86, 526.

17. R. H. Stretch, J. D. Vail, and J. P. Mahoney (1985), "Posttraumatic Stress Disorder Among Army Nurse Corps Vietnam Veterans," *Journal of Consulting and Clinical Psychology* 53, 704–08.

18. American Psychiatric Association, op. cit., p. 380.

19. M. J. Horowitz (1986), *Stress Response Syndromes,* 2nd ed. (New York: Aronson), pp. 1–42.

20. M. J. Horowitz, N. Wilner, and W. Alvarez, (1979), "Impact of Event Scale: A Measure of Subjective Stress," *Psychosomatic Medicine* 41, 209–18.

21. J. P. Wilson, W. K. Smith, and S. K. Johnson (1985), "A Comparative Analysis of PTSD Among Various Survivor Groups," in C. Figley (ed.), op. cit., pp. 142–72. R. M. Scurfield, (1985), "Post-Trauma Stress Assessment and Treatment: Overview and Formulations," in Ibid., pp. 219–56.

22. L. L. Dock and I. M. Stewart (1932), *A Short History of Nursing: From the Earliest Times to the Present Day,* 3rd ed. (New York: Putnam), pp. 351, 358.

23. V. Brittain, op. cit., p. 470.

24. C. Dewane (1984), "Posttraumatic Stress Disorder in Medical Personnel in Vietnam," *Hospital and Community Psychiatry* 35, 1232–34.

25. M. J. Horowitz op. cit., pp. 57–59.

26. W. Smith (1983, October 31), "Carnage in Lebanon," *Time* 122, pp.14–19.

27. B. L. Green, J. P. Wilson, and J. D. Lindy, (1985), "Conceptualizing Post-Traumatic Stress Disorder: A Psychosocial Framework," in C. R. Figley, op. cit., pp. 63–66.

28. C. R. Figley, op. cit.

29. A. Egendorf et al., op. cit.

Chapter 13: Lessons Learned from the War

1. B. Hoey (1984, April), "When Nurses Go to 'War'," *Airman,* 25–30.

Chapter 14: Conclusions

1. E. A. Paul (1985), "Wounded Healers: A Summary of the Vietnam Nurses Veterans Project," *Military Medicine* 150, 571–76. J. Schnaier (1982), "Women Vietnam Veterans and Their Mental Health Adjustment: A Study of Their Experience and Post-Traumatic Stress," unpublished master's thesis, University of Maryland.

2. *War Nurse: The True Story of a Woman Who Lived, Loved and Suffered on the Western Front* (1930) (New York: Cosmopolitan Book Corporation). A. Harrison (ed.) (1944), *Gray and Scarlet: Letters from the War Areas by Army Sisters on Active Duty* (London: Hodder & Stoughton). B. McBryde (1979), *A Nurse's War* (New York: Universe Books). T. Archard (1945), *G.I. Nightingale: The Story of an American Army Nurse* (New York: W. W. Norton).

3. V. Brittain (1933, reprinted 1978), *Testament of Youth* (London: Virago Books), p.291.

4. J. Mackinnon (1987, May 23), "Women are War Veterans, Too," *Newport Daily News,* pp. 1, 12. P. Earley (1982, February), "Nurses Haunted by Memories of Service in Vietnam," *The American Nurse,* p. 8. E. Obergon (1988, May 29), "Vietnam Nurses: Memorial Day Sharpens Vivid Images of a Devastating Era," *Austin American Statesman,* E1, E12. V. French-Lankarge (1988, November 11), "The Women of the War," *Hampshire Life,* 6–10, 54. "Women Vets Need Help," (1987, October), *VFW* 24–25, 60.

5. *Nurse: Vietnam Veterans Memorial Project* (1983), brochure available from Vietnam Nurse Memorial Project, 511 Eleventh Avenue South, Box 45, Minneapolis, MN 55415. There are two memorials—one planned, the other located in New Hampshire—that honor all women who served in the military. Information about these tributes can be found in *The Memorial Bell Tower: A National Tribute to all American Women Who Sacrificed Their Lives in the Wars of Our Country,* Booklet available from Memorial Bell Tower, Cathedral in the Pines, Rindge, NH, and *Women in Military Service Memorial,* Booklet available from Women in Military Service Memorial, P.O. Box 560, Washington, DC, 20042-0560.

References

Adler, A. (1943). "Neuropsychiatric Complaints of Victims of Boston's Coconut Grove Fire."*Journal of the American Medical Association* 123:1098–11.

Ahart, G. J. (1982). *Actions Needed to Insure That Female Veterans Have Equal Access to VA Benefits*. GAO/HRD-82-98. Report to Senator Inouye. Washington, DC: General Accounting Office, September.

American Nurses Association (1967). *Facts About Nursing: A Statistical Summary—1967 Edition*. New York: American Nurses Association.

"American Nurses Association's First Position on Education in Nursing" (1966). *American Journal of Nursing* 66: 515–17.

American Psychiatric Association (1980). *Diagnostic and Statistical Manual of Mental Disorders*. 3d ed. Washington, DC: APA.

Archard, T. (1945). *G.I. Nightingale: The Story of an American Army Nurse*. New York: W. W. Norton.

Archibald, H. C., Long, D. M., and Miller, C. (1962). "Gross Stress Reaction in Combat: A 15-Year Follow-Up." *American Journal of Psychiatry* 119: 317–21.

"Army Loses Doctor and Two Nurses in Vietnam" (1966). News release from Office of the Surgeon General, U.S. Army, Technical Liaison Division, Washington, DC, February 28.

"Army Nurse Awarded DAR Medal Posthumously" (1970). News release from Office of the Surgeon General, U.S. Army, Technical Liaison Division, Washington, DC, April 27.

"Army Nurse Killed by Enemy Rocket " (1969). *Army Reporter* (June 23) 1.

Baker, M. (1981). *Nam.* New York: Quill.

Baker, R. R., Menard, S., Johns, L., Rhoads, J., and Denny, N. (1987). "Female Army Nurses Assigned to Vietnam: Personal and Professional Impact." Paper presented at the 95th Annual Convention of the American Psychological Association, New York, August.

Blank, A. S. (1982). "The Stresses of War: The Example of Vietnam." In L. Goldberger and S. Breznitz (eds.), *Handbook of Stress: Theoretical and Clinical Aspects*, pp.631–43. New York: Free Press.

Borus, J. F. (1974). "Incidence of Maladjustment in Vietnam Returnees." *Archives of General Psychiatry* 30: 554–57.

Boulanger, G. (1981). "Changes in Stress Reaction over Time." In *Legacies of Vietnam: Comparative Adjustments of Veterans and Their Peers*. Report to the 97th Congress, first session. House Committee Print Number 14.

Bourne, P. G. (1970). *Men, Stress, and Vietnam.* Boston: Little, Brown.

Bowers, B. (1987). "Women Vets Fighting to Keep Monument Hope Alive." *Plainfield Courier News*, November 9, 1.

Braverman, M. (1980). "Onset of Psychotraumatic Reactions." *Journal of Forensic Science* 4: 821–25.

Brett, E. A., and Hartman, C. R. (1985). "Imagery and Posttraumatic Stress Disorder: An Overview." *American Journal of Psychiatry* 142: 417–24.

Breuer, J. & Freud, S. (1955). *Studies in Hysteria.* Standard edition. London: Hogarth Press (originally published 1895).

Brittain, V. (1933, reprinted 1978). *Testament of Youth.* London: Virago Books.

—— (1957, reprinted 1981). *Testament of Experience.* New York: Seaview Books.

Brody, J. (1982). "Remembering the Hyatt Disaster: Emotional Scars Persist a Year Later." *New York Times* (July 6), pp. 1, 6.

Caplan, G., & Killilea, M. (eds.) (1976). *Support Systems and Mutual Help: Multidisciplinary Explorations.* New York: Grune & Stratton.

Carnegie, M. E. (1984). "Black Nurses at the Front." *American Journal of Nursing* 84: 1250–52.

Chamberlin, B. C. (1980). "Mayo Seminars in Psychiatry: The Psychological Aftermath of Disaster." *Journal of Clinical Psychiatry* 41: 238–44.

Coppola, V. (1984). "They Also Served." *Newsweek,* November 12, 35–36.

Crabb, M. (1981). "School Mental Health Services Following an Environmental Disaster." *Journal of School Health* 51: 165–67.

Curtis, D. E. (1984). "The Way It Was." *American Journal of Nursing* 84, 1253–54.

Daly, R. J. (1983). Samuel Pepys and Post-Traumatic Stress Disorder." *British Journal of Psychiatry* 143, 64–68.

Decorations and Awards. Army regulations 672-5-2 July 1967 and 672-5-1 April 1984. Washington, DC: U.S. Government Printing Office.

DeFazio, V. J., Rustin, M., and Diamond, A. (1975). "Symptom Development in Vietnam-Era Veterans." *American Journal of Orthopsychiatry* 45, 158–63.

Dewane, C. (1984). "Posttraumatic Stress Disorder in Medical Personnel in Vietnam." *Hospital and Community Psychiatry* 35, 1232–34.

Dock, L. L. and Stewart, I. M. (1932). *A Short History of Nursing: From the Earliest Times to the Present day.* 3d edition. New York: Putnam.

Dougan, C., and Lipsman, S. (1984). *The Vietnam Experience: A Nation Divided.* Boston: Boston Publishing Company.

Dougan, C., and Weiss, S. (1984). *The Vietnam Experience: Nineteen Sixty-Eight.* Boston: Boston Publishing Company.

Dullea, G. (1981). "Women Speaking Out on Effects of Duty in Vietnam." *New York Times,* (March 23), pp. 1, 13.

Durr, E. (1987). "Vietnam Experience Shaped Nurse's Life." *Watertown Daily Times* (January 19), p.9.

Earley, P. (1982). "Nurses Haunted by Memories of Service in Vietnam." *American Nurse,* February 8.

Eaton, W. W., Segal, J. J., and Weinfeld, M. (1981). "Impairment in Holocaust Survivors After 33 Years: Data from an Unbiased Community Sample." *American Journal of Psychiatry* 139: 773–77.

Edelman, B. (ed.) (1986). *Dear America: Letters Home from Vietnam.* New York: Pocket Books.

Egendorf, A., Kadushin, C., Laufer, R., Rothbart, G., and Sloan, L. (1981). In *Legacies of Vietnam: Comparative Adjustments of Veterans and Their Peers.* Vols. 1–5. Report to the 97th Congress, first session. House Committee Print Number 14, March.

Elvenstar, D. (1980). Mary Comes Marching Home. *California Living, Los Angeles Herald Examiner,* December 14, 5–10, 21.

Enzie, R. F., Sawyer, R. N., and Montgomery, F. A. (1973). "Manifest Anxiety of Vietnam Returnees and Undergraduates." *Psychological Reports* 33: 446–50.

Figley, C. R. (ed.) (1978). *Stress Disorders Among Vietnam Veterans: Theory, Research, and Treatment.* New York: Brunner/Mazel.

——— (ed.) (1985). *Trauma and Its Wake: The Study and Treatment of Post-Traumatic Stress Disorder.* New York: Brunner/Mazel.

"First Nurse Killed in Action in Vietnam " (1969). News release from Office of the Surgeon General, U.S. Army, Technical Liaison Division, Washington, DC, June 13.

Fisher, B. (1983). "The Nurses Who Died in Vietnam, *Fort Worth Star-Telegram,* May 29, pp. D1, D5.

Fitzgerald, F. (1972). *Fire in the Lake: The Vietnamese and the Americans in Vietnam.* Boston: Atlantic/Little, Brown.

Frank, A. (1984). "A Nurse Under Fire: Jersey City Woman Recalls Heat of Battle." *Star Ledger,* June 7, pp.1, 22.

Frank, M. E. and Piemonte, R. V. (1985). "The Army Nurse Corps: A Decade of Change." *American Journal of Nursing* 85, 985–88.

Freedman, D. (1984):"Women at War." *San Antonio Light,* August 19, 15–23.

Freedman, D., and Rhoads, J. N. (1987). *Nurses in Vietnam: The Forgotten Warriors.* Austin, TX: Texas Monthly Press.

French-Lankarge, V. (1988). "The Women of the War." *Hampshire Life,* November 11, 6–10, 54.

Frye, J. S., and Stockton, R. A. (1982). "Discriminant Analysis of PTSD Among a Group of Vietnam Veterans." *American Journal of Psychiatry* 139, 52–56.

Furey, J. (1982). "For Some the War Rages On." *American Journal of Nursing* 82, 1695–96.

Furey, J. (1983). "The Walk to the Wall." Unpublished poem.

Gilbert, L. (producer). September 1972 to February 1983. "M*A*S*H" [television series].

Gilligan, C. (1983). *In a Different Voice: Psychological Theory and Women's Development.* Cambridge, MA: Harvard University Press.

Glasser, R. J. (1971). *365 Days.* New York: Braziller.

Goleman, D. (1985). "Emotional Impact of disaster: Sense of Benign World is Lost." *New York Times,* November 26, C1, C6.

Goodman, R. (1985). *Queensland Nurses: Boer War to Vietnam.* Brisbane: Boolarong Publications.

Gray, J. G. (1970). *The Warriors: Reflections on Men in Battle.* New York: Harper & Row.

Green, B. L. (1982). "Assessing Levels of Psychological Impairment Following Disaster: Consideration of Actual and Methodological Dimensions." *Journal of Nervous and Mental Disease* 170, 544–52.

Green, B. L., Wilson, J. P., and Lindy, J. D. (1985). "Conceptualizing Post-Traumatic Stress Disorder: A Psychosocial Framework." In C. R. Figley (ed.), *Trauma and Its Wake: The Study and Treatment of Post-Traumatic Stress Disorder,* pp.53–69. New York: Brunner/Mazel.

Grinker, R. R., and Spiegel, J. P. (1945). *Men Under Stress.* Philadelphia: Blakiston.

Grunwald, D. (1981). "Crying Need." *Parade Magazine,* August 23, 12–13.

Haber, J., Leach, A., Schudy, S., and Sideleau, B. (1982). *Comprehensive Psychiatric Nursing.* 2d ed. New York: McGraw-Hill.

Halloran, R. (1986). "Women, Blacks, Spouses Transforming the Military." *New York Times,* August 25, 1, 14.

Harris, L. (1980). *Myths and Realities: A Study of Attitudes Toward Vietnam Era Veterans.* Washington, DC: U.S. Government Printing Office.

Harrison, A. (ed.) (1944). *Gray and Scarlet: Letters from the War Areas by Army Sisters on Active Duty.* London: Hodder & Stoughton.

Hess, E. (1986). "Statue of Limitation?" *Village Voice,* July 15, 74.

Higonnet, M. R. and Higonnet, P. L. R. (1987). "The Double Helix." In Higonnet, M. R., Jenson, J., Michel, S., and Weitz, M. C. (eds.), *Behind the Lines: Gender and the Two World Wars,* pp.31–51. New Haven, CT: Yale University Press.

Higonnet, M. R., Jenson, J., Michel, S., and Weitz, M. C. (eds.) (1987). *Behind the Lines: Gender and the Two World Wars.* New Haven, CT: Yale University Press.

Hocking, F. (1970). "Psychiatric Aspects of Extreme Environmental Stress." *Diseases of the Nervous System* 31:524–45.

Hoey, B. (1984). "When Nurses Go to 'War'." *Airman,* April, 25–30.

Holm, J. (1982). *Women in the Military: An Unfinished Revolution.* Novato, CA: Presidio Press.

Horne, A. D. (ed.). (1981). *The Wounded Generation: America After Vietnam.* Englewood Cliffs, NJ: Prentice Hall.

Horowitz, M. J. (1982). "Stress Response Syndromes and Their Treatment." In L. Goldberger and S. Breznitz (eds.), *Handbook of Stress: Theoretical and Clinical Aspects.* New York: Free Press.

Horowitz, M. J. (1986). *Stress Response Syndromes.* 2d ed. New York: Aronson.

Horowitz, M. J., and Solomon, G. (1975). "Prediction of Delayed Stress Response Syndrome in Vietnam Veterans." *Journal of Social Issues* 31, 67–79.

Horowitz, M. J., Wilner, N., and Alvarez, W. (1979). "Impact of Event Scale: A Measure of Subjective Stress." *Psychosomatic Medicine* 41, 209–18.

Horowitz, M. J., Wilner, N., Kaltreider, N., and Alvarez, W. (1980). Signs and Symptoms of Post-Traumatic Stress Disorder." *Archives of General Psychiatry* 37, 85–92.

Hudak, C., Gallo, B., and Lohr, T. (1986). *Critical Care Nursing.* 4th ed. Philadelphia: Lippincott.

Humle, C. (1956). *A Nun's Story.* Boston: Little, Brown.

Janoff-Bulman, R. (1985). "The Aftermath of Victimization: Rebuilding Shattered Assumptions." In C. Figley (ed.), *Trauma and Its Wake: The Study and Treatment of Post-Traumatic Stress Disorder,* pp.15–35. New York: Brunner/Mazel.

Kalisch, P. A., and Kalisch, B. J. (1976). "Nurses Under Fire: The World War II Experiences of Nurses on Bataan and Corregidor." *Nursing Research* 25, 409–28.

———— (1986). *The Advance of American Nursing.* 2d edition. Boston: Little, Brown.

———— (1987). *The Changing Image of the Nurse.* Menlo Park, CA: Addison-Wesley.

Kalisch, P. A. and Scobey, M. (1983). "Female Nurses in American Wars." *Armed Forces and Society* 9, 215–44.

Kardiner, A., and Speigel, H. (1947). *War, Stress, and Neurotic Illness.* New York: Hoeber.

Karnow, S. (1983). *Vietnam: A History.* New York: Viking Press.

Kirk, D. (1965). "It was 2:00 A.M. Saigon Time." *American Journal of Nursing* 65, 77–79.

Kneisl, C. R., and Ames, S. W. (1986). *Adult Health Nursing: A Biopsychosocial Approach.* Menlo Park, CA: Addison-Wesley.

Kolb, L. C. (1986). "Post-Traumatic Stress Disorder in Vietnam Veterans." *New England Journal of Medicine* 314, 641–42.

Krippendorf, K. (1980). *Content Analysis: An Introduction to Its Methodology.* London: Sage Publications.

Krupnick, J. L., and Horowitz, M. J. (1981). "Stress Response syndromes: Recurrent Themes." *Archives of General Psychiatry* 38, 428–35.

Laufer, R. F., Yager, T., Frey-Wouters, E., and Donnellan, J. (1981). "Post-War Trauma: Social and Psychological Problems of Vietnam Veterans in the Aftermath of the Vietnam War." In A. Egendorf, C. Kadushin, R. Laufer, G. Rothbart, and L. Sloan (eds.), *Legacies of Vietnam: Comparative Adjustments of Veterans and Their Peers,* 313–473 (Report to the 97th Congress, first session. House Committee Print Number 14.

Lifton, R. J. (1968). *Death in Life.* New York: Random House.

———— (1973). *Home from the War.* New York: Simon and Schuster.

Lindemann, E. (1944). "Symptomatology and Management of Acute Grief." *American Journal of Psychiatry* 101, 141–48.

Lynaugh, J., and Fagin, C. (1988). "Nursing Comes of Age." *Image: Journal of Nursing Scholarship* 20, Winter, 181–90.

Mackinnon, J. (1987), "Women are War Veterans, Too." *Newport Daily News,* May 23, 1, 12.

MacPherson, M. (1984). "Vietnam Nurses: These are the Women Who Went to War." *Ms. Magazine* June, 52–55, 104–105.

———— (1985). *Long Time Passing: Vietnam and the Haunted Generation.* New York: Doubleday.

Mann, J. (1983), "They Also Serve." *Washington Post,* March, 1.

Marshall, K. (1987). *In the Combat Zone: An Oral History of American Women in Vietnam.* Boston: Little, Brown.

May, A. (1983). *Witness to War: A biography of Marguerite Higgins.* New York: Beaufort Books.

McBryde, B. (1979). *A Nurse's War.* New York: Universe Books.

McCaughey, B. G. and Garrick, J. (1987). "Naval Support Activity

Hospital Da Nang Combat Casualty Deaths January to June 1968."
Military Medicine 152, 284–89.

McKay, B. (1968). "Civilian Assignment." *American Journal of Nursing* 68, 336–338.

McVicker, S. (1985), "Invisible Veterans: The Women Who Served in Vietnam." *Journal of Psychosocial Nursing* 23, 12–19.

——— (1987). "Vietnam." *NSNA/Imprint* 34, 42–45.

Menninger, W. C. (1947). "Psychiatric Experience in the War, 1941–1946." *American Journal of Psychiatry* 103, 577–86.

Mithers, C. (1984). "Picking Up the Pieces." *Village Voice,* May 29, 21–23, 42.

Mott, F. W. (1919). *War Neuroses and Shell Shock.* London: Oxford Medical Publications.

"Much Too Macho: Sexist Treatment in the Navy and Marines " (1987). *Time,* 130, September 28, p.28.

Myers, C. S. (1940). *Shell Shock in France 1914–1918.* Cambridge: Cambridge University Press.

Nace, E. P., O'Brien, C. P., Mintz, J., Ream, N., and Meyers, A. (1978). "Adjustment Among Vietnam Veteran Drug Users Two Years Post-Service." In C. R. Figley (ed.), *Stress Disorders Among Vietnam Veterans: Theory, Research, Treatment.* New York: Brunner/Mazel.

Neel, S. (1973). *Medical Support of the U.S. Army in Vietnam, 1965–1970.* Department of the Army Publication No. 008-029-00088-1. Washington, DC: U.S. Government Printing Office.

Neiderland, W. G. (1964). "Psychiatric Disorders Among Persecution Victims: A Contribution to the Understanding of Concentration Camp Pathology and Its Aftereffects." *Journal of Nervous and Mental Disease* 139, 458–74.

Nordheimer, J. (1971). "Medal of Honor Winner Dies." *New York Times,* May 26, 1.

Norman, E. (1982). "The Victims Who Survived." *American Journal of Nursing* 82, 1696–98.

——— (1986a). "Nurses in War: A Study of Female Military Nurses Who Served in Vietnam During the War Years 1965–1973." Unpublished doctoral dissertation. New York University.

——— (1986b). "A Study of Female Military Nurses in Vietnam During the War Years 1965–1973." *Journal of Nursing History* 2, 43–60.

——— (1988). "Post-Traumatic Stress Disorder in Military Nurses Who Served in Vietnam During the War Years 1965–1973." *Military Medicine* 153, 238–42.

——— (1989). "The Wartime Experience of Military Nurses in Vietnam, 1965–1973." *Western Journal of Nursing Research* 11, 219–33.

Nurse: Vietnam Veterans Memorial Project. (1983). Brochure available from Vietnam Nurse Memorial Project, 511 Eleventh Avenue South, Box 45, Minneapolis, Minnesota, 55415.

"Nurses Dispute and Defend Memoir on Life in Vietnam War " (1985). *New York Times,* February 12, p. 20.

Obergon, E. (1988). "Vietnam Nurses: Memorial Day Sharpens Vivid Images of a Devastating Era." *Austin American Statesman,* May 29, E1, E12.

Odom, J. D. (1986). "The Vietnam Nurses Can't Forget." *American Journal of Nursing* 86, 1035–37.

O'Neill, L. D. (ed.) (1979). *The Women's Book of World Records and Achievements.* New York: Doubleday.

Paul, E. A. (1985). "Wounded Healers: A Summary of the Vietnam Nurses Veterans Project." *Military Medicine* 150, 571–76.

Paul, E., and O'Neill, J. (1986). "American Nurses in Vietnam: Stressors and Aftereffects." *American Journal of Nursing* 86, 526.

Redmond, J. (1943). *I Served on Bataan.* Philadelphia: J. B. Lippincott.

Reverby, S. (1987). *Ordered to Care: The Dilemma of American Nursing.* New York: Cambridge University Press.

Rice-Grant, S. K. (1986). "Does Anyone Care: About the Health Problems of Women Who Served in Vietnam." Unpublished master's thesis, California State University, Sacramento.

Rogers, B., & Nickolaus, J. (1987). "Psychological Issues of Vietnam Veteran Nurses." *Journal of Psychosocial Nursing* 25, 220–25.

Rustad, M. (1982). *Women in Khaki: The American Enlisted Woman.* New York: Praeger.

Sandrich, M. (director) (1943). *So Proudly We Hail* (Film). Hollywood, California: Paramount.

Santoli, A. (1981). *Everything We Had.* New York: Random House.

Saywell, S. (1985). *Women in War: First-Hand Accounts from World War II to El Salvador.* New York: Viking.

Schlesinger, A. M. (ed.) (1983). *The Almanac of American History.* New York: Putnam.

Schnaier, J. (1982). "Women Vietnam Veterans and Their Mental Health Adjustment: A Study of Their Experience and Post-Traumatic Stress." Unpublished master's thesis, University of Maryland.

Scurfield, R. M. (1985). "Post-Trauma Stress Assessment and Treatment: Overview and Formulations." In C. Figley (ed.), *Trauma and its Wake: The Study and Treatment of Post-Traumatic Stress Disorder,* pp.219–56. New York: Brunner/Mazel.

Shea, F. (1983). "Stress of Caring for Combat Casualties." *U.S. Navy Medicine,* January–February, 4–7.

Shipler, D. K. (1983). "The Other Israeli Casualties: The Mentally Scarred." *New York Times,* January, 2.

Smith, D. (1979). "Women in the Military." In L. O'Neill (ed.), *The Women's Book of World Records and Achievements.* New York: Doubleday.

Smith, W. (1983). "Carnage in Lebanon." *Time* 122, October 31, 14–19.

Spelts, D. (1986). "Nurses Who Served—and Who Did Not Return." *American Journal of Nursing* 86, 1037–39.

Spooner Schwartz, L. (1988) "Women and the Vietnam Experience." *Image: Journal of Nursing Scholarship* 19, 168–73.

Strange, J. M. (1987). *Shock Trauma Care Plans*. Springhouse, PA: Springhouse.

Strayer, R., and Ellenhorn, L. (1973). "Vietnam Veterans: A Study Exploring Adjustment Patterns and Attitudes." *Journal of Social Issues* 31, 81–94.

Stretch, R. H., Vail, J. D., and Mahoney, J. P. (1985). "Posttraumatic Stress Disorder Among Army Nurse Corps Vietnam Veterans." *Journal of Consulting and Clinical Psychology* 53, 704–708.

Sturm, T. R. (1977). "By Death Undaunted." *Airman*, May, 25–30.

Tamerious, R. K. (1988). Viet Nam—A Legacy of Healing." *California Nursing Review* 10(5), 14–17, 34–38, 44–48.

The Memorial Bell Tower: A National Tribute to All American Women Who Sacrificed Their Lives in the Wars of Our Country. Booklet available from Memorial Bell Tower, Cathedral in the Pines, Rindge, NH.

Theiler, P. (1984). "A Vietnam Aftermath: The Untold Story of Women and Agent Orange." *Common Cause Magazine*, November/December, 29–34.

Ullom, M. (n.d.). *The Philippine Assignment: Some Aspects of the Army Nurse Corps in the Philippine Islands 1940–1945*. Unpublished manuscript. Department of the Army, Center of Military History, Washington, DC.

United States Department of Health and Human Services (1986). *Report on Nursing. Fifth Report to the President and Congress on the Status of Health Personnel in the U.S*. DHHS publication no. 0906804. Washington, DC: U.S. Government Printing Office.

Van Devanter, L. and Morgan, C. (1983). *Home Before Morning: The Story of an Army Nurse in Vietnam*. New York: Beaufort.

"Vietnam Veteran Nurses Remember Their Past " (1985). *American Journal of Nursing* 85, 1293.

Veterans Administration: Annual Report 1981 (1981). Washington, DC: Veterans Administration (VA 1:1:981).

Walker, J. I. (1981). "The Psychological Problems of Vietnam Veterans." *JAMA* 246, 781–82.

Walker, K. (1983). "The Forgotten Vets." *San Francisco Sunday Examiner & Chronicle*, September 15, 4–5, 7–8, 10.

——— (1985). *A Piece of my Heart: The Stories of 26 American Women Who Served in Vietnam*. Novato, CA: Presidio Press.

War Nurse: The True Story of a Woman Who Lived, Loved, and Suffered on the Western Front (1930). New York: Cosmopolitan Book Corporation.

Weintraub, S. (1976). *War in the Wards*. Novato, CA: Presidio Press.

Wells, H. (1943). *Cherry Ames: Student Nurse.* New York: Grosset and Dunlap.

―――― (1944). *Cherry Ames: Army Nurse.* New York: Grosset and Dunlap.

"What Vietnam Did To Us" (1981). *Newsweek,* December 19, 46–49.

Williams, D. (1985). *To the Angels.* San Francisco: Denson Press.

Wilson, J. P. (1980). "Conflict, Stress and Growth: The Effects of War on Psychological Development Among Vietnam Veterans." In C. R. Figley and S. Leventman (eds.), *Strangers at Home: Vietnam Veterans Since the War.* New York: Praeger.

Wilson, J. P., Smith, W. K., and Johnson, S. K. (1985). "A Comparative Analysis of PTSD Among Various Survivor Groups. In C. Figley (ed.), *Trauma and Its Wake: The Study and Treatment of Post-Traumatic Stress Disorder,* pp.142–72. New York: Brunner/Mazel.

Women in Military Service Memorial. Booklet available from Women in Military Service Memorial, P.O. Box 560, Washington, DC, 20042–0560.

"Women Vets Need Help " (1987). *VFW,* October, 24–25, 60.

"Women Vets Profiled in New VA Study " (1985). *VVA Veteran* 5, October, 6.

Woodham-Smith, C. (1951). *Florence Nightingale: 1820–1910.* New York: McGraw-Hill.

"17 Women Serving on Hospital Ship " (1966). *New York Times,* February 21, 27.

Index

Store use only: 629147

Customer Name: estep, laura
Day Phone: (574) 353-7354
Night Phone:
Fax Number:

Cust Comments :

Order Comments :